D0792627

The Educational Resource Library Asks that you
please return your library materials when you are
done with them. If they have been helpful to you,
they will help another. If you would like to
purchase this title, please contact the librarian and
she can assist you with your purchase.
This Library copy is not for sale.

 Vail Valley Medical Center

RECOVERING FROM MORTALITY

RECOVERING FROM MORTALITY

. . . .

Essays from a Cancer Limbo Time

DEBORAH CUMMING

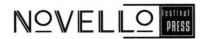

NOVELLO FESTIVAL PRESS 2005

Copyright © 2005 by Robert Cumming

All rights reserved under International and
Pan-American Copyright Conventions.
Published in the United States by
NOVELLO FESTIVAL PRESS,
Charlotte, North Carolina.

Library of Congress Cataloging-in-Publication Data

Cumming, Deborah.
 Recovering from mortality : essays from a cancer limbo time / by
Deborah Cumming ; introduction by Robert Cumming, with an
epilogue by Gabriel Cumming.
    p. cm.
 ISBN 0-9760963-3-1 (trade paper)
 1. Cumming, Deborah—Health. 2. Lungs—Cancer—Patients—
Biography. 3. Metastasis. 4. Terminally ill—Biography. I. Title.
 RC280.L8C845 2005
 362.196'99424'0092—dc22
                        2005001070

Book design by Bonnie Campbell
Printed in the United States of America
FIRST EDITION

Qu'on ne nous raconte pas d'histoires. Qu'on ne nous dise pas du condamné à mort: "Il va payer sa dette à la société", mais: "on va lui couper le cou." Ca n'a l'air de rien. Mais ca fait une petite différence. Et puis, il y a des gens qui préfèrent regarder leur destin dans les yeux.

(Let's not make up stories. Let's not say about the person condemned to death, "He's going to pay his debt to society," but rather, "His throat will be cut." That may seem inconsequential. But it does make a little difference. And after all, some people choose to look their destiny in the eyes.)

—ALBERT CAMUS, "Entre Oui et Non" ("Between Yes and No")

CONTENTS

· ·

INTRODUCTION

· ·

AT THE TIME when Deborah Cumming wrote *Recovering from Mortality,* she was living in a situation not widely recognized but shared by many people. She knew that she might die soon, yet she was not dying now. What is a person to think about in this "limbo" time? How is a person to act? Rather than accept formulaic answers—psychiatric or religious—to these questions, Deborah decided to discover her own path. She didn't want to pass on *her* answers to others—she didn't believe she knew universal answers. She was not interested in adding another story of a cancer patient who survived heroically or who died movingly. Nor did she think she had step-by-step techniques to help with illness or with dying. She did want to commune with others in limbo—with people who, like her, might find it a lonely or mysterious condition, with special darknesses and illuminations. And as she went deeper into the writing, she felt increasingly that she was talking about the human situation in general, since—whether we acknowledge it or not—all our lives will end in the not-very-distant future. She felt that she wanted to be in communication, not only with the dying, but with the living who are ready to acknowledge their mortality.

AUGUST 13, 2000, was a cloudless day, cooler than usual for the Carolinas. Deborah and I had just left our son Gabriel and his bicycle partner in the foothills of the Blue Ridge Mountains.

On the way home we'd decided to climb Crowders Mountain, west of Charlotte. The trails rise about 800 feet. Halfway up Deborah said, "I'm out of breath." We'd taken the steeper, more rocky route; still, this was not rougher than other hikes we were used to. Yet Deborah was gulping for breath, her heartbeat feathery and fast. We turned back.

At two the next morning, she woke with chest pain. Deborah wasn't doctor-prone; ordinarily she preferred other remedies first. "We need to call 911 now," she said.

For a week her general doctor and a heart specialist wavered between several explanations of short breath and the fluid around her heart. Then Deborah spotted on her hospital table an x-ray reading which—mistakenly—had not been passed on to the doctors. It noted a cloudy area on her right lung. Her cardiologist, upset by the hospital oversight, sent her for further radiography and a lung specialist appointment. Two weeks later we knew she probably had a disease we'd had no warning of—lung cancer. After more tests, including a bone biopsy, a diagnosis came: non-small-cell lung cancer, stage IV. "Stage IV" were words even more weighted, we discovered, than "lung cancer": they meant the cancer had spread from lungs to spine—and might be expected to continue to spread. For patients with this disease, average life expectancy was six months. Describing our reactions in the essay called "Slow Shock," Deborah says, *We skipped over treatment and miracles, and went straight to death.*

For the next two years Deborah recorded—not the details of her disease—but her thoughts, feelings, and interactions with other people, in a period when she knew she might die any time. This recording became the source for the essays in *Recovering from Mortality.*

During these years her life was complex. Her father died a fortnight after her first signs of illness. She waded into the duties of settling his estate. She continued to work on housing for low-income citizens of Davidson. Many friends visited, from Davidson and far away; three cherished college classmates came to be with her for a week. She had a strong desire to complete a novel, and to edit her stories, poems and journals. As we became more aware that doctors had no cures for nor certainties about advanced lung cancer—that *we* would have to decide whether taking experimental drugs was worth potential drastic side effects—she entered the search, by Internet and phone and interview, for some reasonable way through the ever-expanding maze of decisions.

In spite of these pursuits—they seemed to multiply as the months continued to unroll without a crisis—she gave a special priority to the essays. Sometimes she wrote in a notebook before getting out of bed in the morning. At night, when I often felt exhausted by the hunt for therapies, she would turn to the computer to go on with the essay in progress. When she finished one she went over it repeatedly, reading it aloud, altering phrases and whole sections to get closer to what she meant. Apart from being with her friends and family, what she wanted to do most before dying was to work on this book.

DEBORAH WAS BORN in Washington, D.C., on June 14, 1941; she grew up in Princeton, New Jersey. Moyne Rice Smith, her mother, had made her way from Oskaloosa, Kansas, to the theatre world of New York, where she appeared in *New Faces of 1935*. After marrying, she became an innovator in dramatics for young people. Blackwell Smith, Deborah's father, whose family had farmed oranges in California, became a New Deal lawyer and lieutenant of Roosevelt. Soon after Deborah was born, he was appointed head of the War Production Board, which assured the supply of materials for the armed forces in World War II. Deborah was surrounded by people who talked politics and art and who, risking major changes in their own lives, saw life as an adventure.

At Swarthmore College she majored in French, graduating with highest honors. Instead of climbing farther in the academic world, she joined the movement for social and economic justice which accompanied the Kennedy-Johnson "War on Poverty." She worked in a bail program for inmates and an Upward Bound program for disadvantaged teenagers in New York. In Washington she wrote reports for the United Planning Organization, which supported community action in low-income neighborhoods. She began to teach—first in India on a "junior" Fulbright fellowship; then, after earning a master's degree at Columbia Teachers College, in a Manhattan middle school. Later she joined me at the City College of New York, in a program designed to make it possible for poorly-prepared and foreign students to succeed there.

One of her gifts as a teacher was the way in which she introduced students to writing about their own lives. She wanted to know about them—more intensely than they expected. They responded by digging into their lives more deeply than typical assignments require. When we moved to teach at Lander College, in a mills-and-farming town in rural South Carolina, Deborah took up her quest in unfamiliar country, asking students for *more* from their consciousness of family, of race, of economic conditions. At the same time she was writing her own poems and stories: she won the South Carolina state fellowship for a fiction writer in 1995-96. When she stopped teaching after twenty years in South Carolina, she expected to focus her life on writing.

THE TIME BETWEEN Deborah's diagnosis and her death seemed to her unlike other periods. She made discoveries—about living and dying, about herself. She made choices, more final than any she'd made before. The discoveries and choices transformed her, she thought, into another kind of person. Her inner changes—and her encounters with people around her—were the basic elements of what she felt to be the most intense, most alive part of her life.

I signed up for a cram course in death and life: I was the student, the teacher, and the subject matter, she writes in the essays. *I have an opportunity for awareness, for learning, for exploration and discovery.* Impermanence—a discovery which occurs at least vaguely to everyone through aging and losses—becomes real in an unexpected way when *your* impermanence can likely be reckoned in weeks. Times of resignation, which may take the forms of depression or detachment, can alternate with moments of euphoria: *I am alive!* Deborah writes. As she became familiar in herself with these extremes of an alternation everyone encounters, she came to see that her "case" was not only an instance of cancer. In the words of Tolstoy's *The Death of Ivan Ilych*—a favorite book which became even more luminous for her as the cancer time continued—"it was not a question of illness, but of life and death."

Deborah knew—from the time of diagnosis on—that she wanted *to make something of this time.* But how? We were given more advice than we could use: to go to Hawaii, to develop trust in God or fate, to let go. Deborah was surrounded by concerned, gifted friends. A respected therapist offered to "guide her on her journey." But finally she decided that—as she says in the essay called "Control"—*I wanted to make my own way.* She chose to inquire into the facts about her illness, rather than to leave them to doctors or others. She chose to think about the likelihood that she might die, instead of adopting a "positive" or brave or naïve idea that she must live. She chose not to wrap herself in nostalgia for the past or in regret for what she might have done differently. *I want to be awake,* she writes.

Deborah and I participated in a retreat led by the meditation teacher Rodney Smith during the summer following her diagnosis. Rodney gave her a phrase—*Where is death in this mo-*

ment?—and asked her to keep it in her mind. This phrase co-incided with Deborah's urge to stay aware, and it became increasingly important to her. Friends sometimes ignored or tiptoed by the probability of her early dying, but for Deborah—as *Recovering from Mortality* shows—it was continually present. At the same time she seemed especially alert to life. People who visited during her last months often remarked on how completely she gave herself to them—their concerns, their ideas. Her attention to nature and to books and pictures, registered in her journals and the essays, was deeply concentrated. The bifocal vision she developed—embracing both facts, that she was dying and living—gave an extraordinary intensity to this part of her life. *We can live only in the moment,* she writes.

Years before she knew she had cancer, Deborah composed a somewhat wry poem addressed to our son Gabriel, titled "One Last List." It gave him instructions about what music he might play if she were dying. *No Romantics,* she says. *Monteverdi. Sitar music. Marian Anderson.* In October, 2002, an MRI scan showed that the cancer had moved to her brain. For the next four months she was able to stay at home as she had hoped, without overwhelming pain. She talked with people close to her and listened to CD's of her favorite Monteverdi and Bach pieces, Indian ragas, and Marian Anderson. She died there on March 10, 2003.

During the preceding August, the last month when she felt her mind to be completely active, she made a complete revision and reorganization of *Recovering from Mortality*, putting the book together as it now exists. She describes her sense of the limbo period. *I was undergoing a transformation. . . . I can make choices. . . . It is death that keeps me alive. . . . I have something to do, to live the life I have. I'm busy with my task. . . .*

—ROBERT CUMMING

PREFACE

. . . .

The first day's quiet. The second; the second
year. I'm taking up my life. If you were here
who I am honest with
I'd have to think a long time
to say the simplest thing:
nothing like anything I know.

—JEAN VALENTINE, "Turn"

THESE ESSAYS WERE written during the limbo time of my cancer, a period that began when I started improving from treatment and ended when the cancer was progressing again. In my case, the limbo time lasted about a year, depending on which calendar markers I use, a surprisingly long time for a person diagnosed with Stage IV lung cancer, one of the cancers still waiting for a medical breakthrough.

Although I wasn't concerned with telling one more cancer story—there are plenty of useful books of this kind—I do refer to events along the way, before and during the limbo time. The cancer experience is a road dotted by little way stations—tests, doctors' visits, blood draws, chemotherapy infusions—leading to a known destination—death—but by an unknown number of perambulations. During the first part of my journey, when I was learning about the diagnosis of metastatic non-small-cell lung cancer, choosing treatment with chemo-therapy and a trial drug called Iressa (or placebo), and passing time in the chemo room, I gave no thought to writing essays. Occasionally, I made entries in my journal, and I talked with my family and friends.

When the chemo treatment was over and I was making significant improvement (possibly because I continued to take the experimental pills), I wanted to explore my thoughts. I had more time to think: less of my energy was going into surviving the disease and the treatment. I was also more able to think: "chemobrain," a mind-dimming side effect of chemotherapy, was clearing off like a misty morning. I realized that I was still undergoing a transformation and now had an opportunity to try to identify and even share it with others in case they might find my experience helpful.

The better you do during the limbo time, the more alone you are. Doctors are most attentive when there's a down-swing. Friends don't want to treat you like an invalid. And yet the cancer may not be gone, may be waiting to re-emerge from the wings, may even now be doing its work while you pretend you've forgotten it. I knew that my kind of cancer was not curable, and yet, for a spell, it seemed to have vanished. Some other cancer patients have reason to believe their cancer has been eradicated, and yet, in their heart of hearts, they are never sure. I noticed that among the many books about cancer—survivors' stories of remarkable recoveries, accounts of loved ones' struggles toward death, guidance for coping and learning—there were few focusing on the limbo time. I thought I might offer companionship to some people in the limbo time and perhaps to others who think about the fascinating, shifting, blurry margin of dying and living.

These essays are forays I made into a territory I'm no longer in. My cancer has progressed and I'm in treatment again. It's a different terrain, not encompassed by this particular collection. As I wrote, I had one primary guideline: I simply tried to be honest. I dedicate what I've written to my husband Bob and my son Gabriel: *you who I am honest with.*

AUGUST 2002

MORTALITY

. . . .

WARNING: The prudent mariner will not rely solely on
any single aid to navigation, particularly on floating aids.

—COAST AND GEODETIC SURVEY NAUTICAL CHART

I AM LUCK

. . . .

I ONCE HAD a student named Rose whose brief autobiography written in the first class of English 100 concluded: *I am luck*. I don't remember whether Rose lasted through the whole semester, but I know she didn't stay in college longer than a year. By many people's standards, her life has probably not been luck. But mine has been.

When I was diagnosed with lung cancer, my luck shifted. *My luck she is running out*, says the fisherman in an old children's tale, whose net no longer fills with fish. Actually, though, I've never felt my luck she is running out. I have continued to feel I am luck.

For one thing, my luck has held pretty steady for sixty years. I guess the not-so-good luck was piling up unnoticed and made itself known all at once. That's what Stage IV cancer is, a pile-up of not-so-good luck. For another thing, I've had the best support imaginable: my totally devoted husband; a son who, at 22, is just the right age to give energy, love, and wit in a steady flow and who happens to be free to live with us; and many friends who have rallied round.

Anyone who has really suffered from cancer will recognize that, so far, I haven't. Some difficulty breathing but not much, some fatigue, some nausea and vomiting from the chemotherapy. Maybe deeper physical suffering will come later, but for now I have been allowed to have an experience of another kind: an opportunity for awareness, for learning, for exploration and discovery.

Several times I've seen the face of someone who knows what lung cancer can be like. My friend the oncology chaplain, who explained that the word *remission* isn't used for lung cancer because it doesn't happen. A hospice director, who, when I said my cancer seemed to be gone, said *maybe it is so, maybe it is so* in a way that conveyed hope, doubt, and the wisdom of experience all at once. These people are thinking of more than the killer statistics for lung cancer; they are thinking also of the suffering they have seen. A cancer phone-friend who now has a second recurrence of metastasized lung cancer tells me of the pain in the vertebrae of her upper back and the pain of having a tube rammed in between her ribs to drain the pleura. I have not had to endure this. All I've had to face is death itself.

Five years ago we moved from a house and woods and fields we loved very much. There was a lot of sorting and packing to be done, but I felt that there was something I had to do first. First I had to gather the photographs, drawings, journal entries, poems the three of us had produced over the years and arrange them in notebooks, to make something of our years there. It took several weeks of full-time work to compile the four volumes. Then I was ready to do the other work of moving.

Almost my first thought after I was told "the average life expectancy is twenty-four weeks" was: I have work to do. I wanted to go through my old journals and letters and throw away the parts that didn't need to be kept beyond my life and organize the rest so others wouldn't have to. I wanted to go through my belongings and my parents', work I felt should be mine. But I didn't even start these tasks. I got caught up in deciding about treatment, doing the treatment, and dealing with people who wished me well. When the chemo was finished and I appeared to be improving, I still wanted to do the clean-up of my life, and I want to still. I want to remember that I haven't done it yet. But first. . . First, I want to make something of this time before it's gone.

Our train may move again any minute now, but there's something I want to say about this station we've paused in before we leave it behind.

SLOW SHOCK

. . . .

ONE SUNDAY MORNING last summer, I was walking through dewy grass down a slight slope in smooth-bottomed flip-flops when I suddenly slipped and fell down. Zip! I felt the nerve communicating from hip to brain. I could hear the nerve jolt in my brain. Almost immediately—but only after these sensations—concepts formed: *I've fallen. I wonder if I'm hurt.* Later more concepts: *Anything can happen in an instant. What you've prepared for isn't what happens.* In an instant I was jarred from hip to brain. But it was an hour later that I felt the shock. I wrote in my journal: "Slow shock. . . possible? Yes."

That was in the pre-cancer time. Today it is six months after I was told I had advanced cancer and, if I was average, I'd have six months to live. I heard the nerve jolt in my brain immediately, but six months later the shock is still registering. Slow shock. Like a time-release pill, the shock will be released through the rest of my life, however long that happens to be.

Rereading the pulmonologist's early notes to my family doctor: "I have no doubt she has metastatic cancer." I feel the shock of seeing it in writing.

A neighbor is surprised I can walk up the road. I protest: "I'm not sick, you know!" Then I remember. "I'm just mortally ill."

I run across the old statistics and feel their shock again: two out of five respond to chemo; without chemo, ten percent live one year; with chemo, two or three more months are added. The oncologist's notes: "She understands there is no cure." I understood there was no cure, that day. But I don't understand it today.

Slow shock. After the pivotal visit with the cardiologist, when we learned that my heart wasn't the main problem, Bob and I drove home by a new route. He was studying the map and directing me through a series of small roads. Our usual interaction: I drove, and he plotted a series of maneuvers no one else had ever tried in order to avoid the main arteries. He asked what the cardiologist said, and turn by turn I told him.

"Take the next left."

"He looked startled when he saw the radiologist's report."

"Now go right for a short distance."

"There are nodules throughout the lungs."

"Two more intersections, then left again."

"And it seems to be in the bones, too."

I wasn't sure he was hearing me. He kept on giving me directions.

We delayed the shock from cardiologist to pulmonologist to bronchoscopy to bone scan to bone biopsy to oncologist.

I remember the two of us lying flat in bed with the light on, like a stone knight and his lady on their sarcophagi, staring ahead toward the bathroom door with the mirror, the bookcase. Six more months to live. We fell all the way down. We thought about death, my death, my scant time to be alive, our scant time to be together. We skipped over treatment and miracles and went straight to death.

LIMBO

. . . .

Nobody, nothing
    ever gave me
        greater thing

than time
    unless light
        and silence

—LORINE NIEDECKER, "Wintergreen Ridge"

THREE MONTHS OR THREE YEARS

. . . .

"How do you know if you are going to die?"
I begged my mother.
We had been traveling for days.
With strange confidence she answered,
"When you can no longer make a fist."

—NAOMI SHIHAB NYE, "Making a Fist"

FINISHING CHEMOTHERAPY AND having a *now-what?* confer-
ence with my doctor has led me into a complex era of mixed,
even contradictory feelings. I wake in the morning uplifted
by the thought that I am free—of chemo; of weekly doctor's
appointments and tests; of certain other obligations—a book
club talk, some visits. I have more time! But how much more
time? Three months to three years, my doctor says, possibly
at random. I'm not free of cancer. And what is that shadowy
new thing in my lung? And why do I feel (somewhat) more
breathless?

I'm free—free to fall back on my own resources. I have to
redefine the challenge. It was easier to face the challenges of
the first phase: to face death, possibly soon; to learn the
rhythm and physical assaults of chemo and blood draws. I
had the help of doctors then, or I had the doctors to be frus-
trated with. Now, post-chemo, I dream that I am talking to
my doctor. I talk on and on, and he finally mutters, "*Som-
meil.*" I'm talking him to sleep.

I send the information about my "very good partial response" to three friends. One says, "Great!" The second says, "I'm sorry." The third, groping carefully, says, "That sounds good, especially in view of the doctor's and your feelings about it." I realize that I can't expect my friends to understand. They could understand when I didn't have long to live. They could understand the debilitation and demoralization of chemo. But what is this shadowy new thing, the very good partial response? I will need to rely less on friends now.

Since I'm feeling more energetic, I'm slipping back into old habits of cleaning, cooking, laundry, bill-paying. I'm returning to old definitions of duty. I amended some of these rules during the time of relative crisis, allowing some things to go undone and others to be shared, learning to ask others to do things and, if I couldn't make myself ask, learning not to be bothered by a smudged kitchen floor. The kitchen floor had often been dirty before—I am not an immaculate housekeeper—but I had always minded. When I thought I was dying, I taught myself to let it go. Now that I'm not dying—am I not dying?—that's harder. And harder to decide whether to resume my recorder group, go back to book club meetings, carry my weight again on the Affordable Housing Coalition board.

For some cancer patients, it is a relief—a joy—to return to normal, to the old cares, to the old activities. And people in the outside world say, "It's so good to see you out and about," just the way they say, "Your hair is coming back!" I'm beginning to repress my vow of honesty. My mother taught me, when I was given a compliment, to just say thank you.

I'm thinking of giving up recorder group, which I rejoined, because of how it has made me worry about cleaning up when they meet at my house. I wrote in my journal:

I want to just hastily pick up and dust and sweep right before they come—not put time and caring into cleaning up. Buy dessert instead of making it. I may have only a few months until I'm ill and in decline, yet I waste precious moments over the questions of what part of the day shall I give to this, how much shall I curtail the urge to clean and just let it be messy or dirty, can I give serious attention to something else and if so what, should I give up recorder group (and other obligations) so I'll stop wasting time over stuff like this and get to what matters to me. . .

When I'm cleaning or trying not to clean, I'm sure I should quit recorder group again. But it's quite different when they are here.

The low level kidding and exchange with R, R, and B; the concentration on playing; the enjoyment of the music we make. I don't know. If I knew it would be three months and not three years, would I quit recorder group?

Old habits, friends, doctors—none of these are now enough. I need to search, I write in my journal, for *deeper sources of resiliency, of strength, of joy.* While most people think I'm returning to a kind of normal, and they have quite appropriately stopped bringing casseroles or sending cards, and when they see me congratulate me on how I look and sometimes on how my "attitude" had brought me through, I'm beginning another leg of the journey. More alone than before, looking for new helpers, learning a new relationship to the questions.

> Oh, MacTavish is dead and his brother don't know it.
> His brother is dead and MacTavish don't know it.
> They're both of them dead
> and both in one bed,
> and neither one knows that the other is dead.
>
> —SCOTTISH SONG

Either we are living or we are dying. I was struck by this state-ment when I read it once in a Buddhist magazine. Bob Dylan said it, too, I think. I believe I get the idea—especially in a song lyric—but when I read it I thought: *No! We are living and we are dying.* At that time, I was already "dying" of cancer but I didn't know it. I knew I was living, and I thought living and dying must be one thing, not an either/or.

"Why do you think you got cancer at this time?" I've been asked. There are problems with this question. For one thing, it assumes there is some kind of "reason" for getting cancer, a reason that is embedded in a prior inner sickness of my own—a moral, an emotional, or a psychological sickness. I have long thought that you're more likely to get a cold if you're run-down or, as my mother used to put it, *under par*—under par in any of a variety of ways. I do believe that stress makes a per-son's health vulnerable. Smoking, of course, is a causal factor, but I hadn't ever smoked. Even if I had, following the line of thought that, in some way, you caused your cancer is a process that is not, as Buddhists say, skillful.

We don't know "why" we got our cancer and we don't know "when," either. A chest x-ray report I never saw suggested the need to "follow" a wispy shadow in my lungs, so I maybe al-ready "had" my cancer as early as 1994, though it didn't an-nounce itself unmistakably until six years later. When that overlooked x-ray was taken, I had just been in a car wreck. Did that trauma suddenly bring on cancer? Two days before my definitive diagnosis this year, my father died. Did that cause my cancer to erupt? A month before that, I climbed a mountain and struggled to breathe. Was that mountain climb the onset of cancer—or was the existing cancer boiling over? If I hadn't climbed that mountain, would the cancer have waited another year perhaps before I knew about it? During all this murky time when I had it but didn't know it, was I living or dying?

Humans love to classify life into stages. The seven ages of man, ladders of moral development, Before and After Christ, "a time to be born and a time to die." There is a time to die, but we only know what it is when the very moment comes. Tolstoy's Ivan Ilych—everyman—is living until he isn't. The moment of his dying, when the onlookers see him in a coma, already checked out, is the moment of most intense living of Ivan's entire life.

Cancer is an insistent opportunity to learn that in dying we are alive, in living we are dying. Even with cancer, it's hard to tell which is which. As Bob and I plunged like high divers into awareness and acceptance of my death, we were also exploring treatment. And so I made the choice to sit in the chemo room lounge chair, swaddled in blankets, with poison dripping into my veins. Sometimes it felt like dying, and it promised only a little more living—at best.

But now I am, the CT report states, *status post chemotherapy*. Should I understand this as status *postpartum* or status *postmortem*? Certain denizens of Dante's world who didn't fit into his system of circles were relegated to Limbo. That's where I am. "The cancer will progress," the doctor wants to make sure I know. "We don't know when. Three months, three years." We talk in terms of "when" the cancer progresses, not "if." I make a careful note of this. I make notes against the possibility of illusion.

THERE ARE MARKERS in our existence. When we pass a certain marker, we are "post." After the moment of giving birth, I was *postpartum*. One day—I don't know when—I will be *postmortem*. These markers—these rare identifiable moments—allow for certain things to happen. *Postpartum* allows for a specific kind of depression. *Postmortem* allows for an autopsy, when the cause of my death can be labeled. I'm post-chemo now. It's almost the only thing I can say for certain. The other thing I can say for certain—I must remind myself—is that a bone biopsy once confirmed that I had adenocarcinoma. The doctor thinks he can say for certain that my cancer is only holding, not gone. A plane in a holding pattern, waiting to be given the go-ahead to land. A caller on hold, waiting to be connected.

I'm not certain even of this. My sister says, "I think of you as healed." A friend reminds me that her ex-husband was supposed to die within three years, and he's "still kicking" thirty years later. A letter from the American Cancer Society begins, "Dear Survivor." Am I healed, still kicking, a survivor?

I look for labels, so I can tell friends what I am. The doctor says, "We don't usually use the word *remission* with lung cancer." He offers me another tag: *very good partial response*. For lung cancer, that's very very good. I went to a school that didn't believe in grading papers with A's and B's. Words were used instead; they were meant to be more human, I suppose, more flexible. But we learned each teacher's system. So I understand my cancer rating to be a *Very Good+*. Fine, but I was always aiming for *Excellent*, or even *Outstanding* or *Superior*. This time I'm happy with *Very Good+*, because not long ago we were looking at a rating I had never thought possible: a *Very Poor* or even—something only other people got—a *Failure*.

ONCE I THOUGHT in months and years. During the chemo time I thought in twenty-one-day units. Now, post-chemo, I think in eight-week units, CT scan to CT scan. I thought the second post-chemo scan would be significant because it would show what happened when the chemicals were no longer mingling with my other body fluids. But the doctor said that no, the next scan after that would tell us more. Maybe he was afraid I'd feel discouraged if the scan showed some disease progression. But it didn't.

I have never had any talent for putting off bad news or good. I've always ripped open the report card or the response to a fellowship application. So after each CT scan I make sure I get the radiologist's report before I hear my doctor's version of it. After picking up the perhaps-more-significant report, I sit in the car in the hospital parking lot, making my way along the rosary beads, words with sanctified meaning in a language no longer spoken—like Latin, Sanscrit, Pali—for which I have no dictionary. *Nonionic. Mediastinum. Hilum. Superolaterally. Post obsructive change. Parenchymal*—three times. *Sclerotic.*

The words seem familiar, but what do they mean?. Looking at an eye chart you recognize the symbols—you've seen them countless times—but is it an 8, a 3, or an S?

I make my way through the report several times. Some words I understand. Those "innumerable" nodules throughout my lungs—the one feature of my cancer story I had really grasped—are now referred to as *minimal, tiny, residual.* The radiologist thinks they may now be only *scarring* and he very scrupulously states that they are "too small to be described as distinct nodules."

AS I TURN OUT of the hospital parking lot, I flick on WDAV, the all-Classical station. Beethoven's Fifth catches me up in its huge paean to life, whirls me with him, past the frustration, anger, and despair that had towed him under, into a vortex of joy in being alive, reasonless joy. Alive! I am alive— I'm going to continue to be alive. Why should I care? I was willing to die, it was all right to die, there was—there is—no reason to cling to life—and yet I'm filled with delight, I'm excited to be given more opportunity for life, I'm grateful for the whole sweep of what I've been given: a chance to learn about death and a chance to come back from it for a while, a chance to live with a greater sense of life. *I am luck!* All my life I've been luck, but I had to tell myself a few months ago that at last my luck had turned, *my luck she was running out.* It seemed only fair, after such a long streak. But now, again, my luck she is running back in. In the drugstore I see Sarah Jetton, who tells me she has prayed for me every night. Thank you, Sarah! In the post office, I see Annie Porges, who would have prayed for me if she had known. Thank you, Annie! Last night I saw Margaret Stauffer, who has me at the top of her prayer list though I didn't know it. Thank you, Margaret! Thank you, luck, for presenting me with Iressa, my trial drug. Now, onward.

I call my doctor. He agrees—I am "*stable*—or better." But it's not like talking to Beethoven's Fifth. I'm an unusual case for him—he has said this before and says it now—and I wish for him, and for me too, that he could experience just a little joy. The cancer ward is filled with people getting sicker, people dying. But I'm not. It's rather fun, for the moment anyway, isn't it?

He is careful to remind me: "The truth is we're going to hear from this again." He says this to explain his hesitancy in referring me, as I request, for my postponed yearly mammogram. He wants to make sure I understand.

"I certainly understand that if I'm dying I don't need to have a mammogram. But it seems to me possible that I'm not dying. Maybe I should do what people who aren't dying do to promote their health, like have a mammogram."

I feel I'm being too harsh with him—using the *D* word—but I can't think of a gentler way to talk about it. It's not about the mammogram. It's about whether I'm living or dying.

· ·

"I shall study deserving."
—EDMUND in *King Lear*

A DEATH SENTENCE, my brother called his cancer. A reprieve, I call this interlude, this lifting of the death sentence. Both sentence and reprieve are randomly administered. I don't smoke, I am a vegetarian. People who know I "lived a clean life," or think they know, express shock at my diagnosis. Are they shocked that I of all people. . . or are they shocked that their fragile structure of goodness and reward is upset? (Anyone who thinks I got what I deserved has kept his views to himself.)

"The Reward of Virtue," the title of a story in my fourth-grade reader, has always stayed with me. A woman who lived alone and was mocked by the neighborhood children stepped on the pointed tines of her rake and punctured her foot. I can still see the row of holes I imagined in the flesh of her sole. One child for some now-forgotten reason decided to be helpful to the unfortunate woman—"virtue"—and earned a reward, I've forgotten what, a pot of gold or a book. To this day I'm careful to lay rakes point downward on the ground, and I assume that virtuous behavior will pay off.

Even when handed a random, undeserved death sentence, one tries to cling to virtue. "There's something different about you," my doctor said now and then during treatment. I felt not just hopeful but proud when he said that, as if my hidden virtue were being glimpsed. Some people like to think that my reprieve is due not only to my lucky trial drug but also—or exclusively—to whatever they value most—my strength of character, my healthy eating habits, or the better-late-than-never intervention of a just God.

Confronted with an arbitrary sentence, most people want to fight it, to reverse it, to do the best work they can to change the outcome. A person who does the most thorough research on the Internet, who is bold to seek out the most expert specialists, has the best chance of winning the race—"the race for the cure." Husbands, especially, eagerly plunge into this work, desperate to take action. Virtue is now not the shield but the sword.

I feel apologetic toward people who want to give me credit for not being felled by the six-month sentence. I didn't try very hard to avoid it. It was my husband, in the way of husbands, who worried about whether we were doing enough research, making enough effort, asking enough questions. He and his close friend, Erwin, who had been a cancer researcher, talked long distance often and lengthily, examining all the angles. I was grateful but especially grateful if their concern enabled me to spend my time in other ways.

If I were falsely accused of a heinous crime, would I not try to hire the best trial lawyer in the land? I don't know. I suppose I would, and I'd use my brain to help him develop the legal case, just as I use my brain now to help develop my medical case. But if I were on death row, I think I would be using some of my energy not to protest the sentence but to accept it. "I have a journey, sir, shortly to go," Kent says after Lear's death, before his own. " My master calls me; I must not say no." From the outset, I felt I had work to do. Certain tasks jumped to the top of the To Do list. And above the practical "set your affairs in order" tasks came the urgent, primordial command to "make your peace with God." I signed up for a cram course in death and life: I was the student, the teacher, and the subject matter. I had to make haste but slowly; whatever time there was—my lifetime—was what I needed; I could not afford distractions such as research into prolonging my life.

Mors janua vitae.
—TOMBSTONE INSCRIPTION

"I believe we all have cancer," a friend said when I told her my diagnosis. An expert on a news program explains that a high percentage of small breast cancers will never progress to the danger stage, an argument against reliance on mammography that reveals more than we need—or, he says, want—to know.

Yes but. . .

Believing that we all have cancer, knowing that one's breasts may be riddled with too-small-to-count cancer cells, realizing that I may have had my present lung cancer for many years before it insisted upon itself: what do I do with such a view of life? It's like the photographs of magnified dust mites, huge monsters with beady eyes and talons that, it turns out, I live with every moment: how should I act on such knowledge?

Really, I want to tell my friend, "getting" cancer is different from your belief that we all have cancer. It was different for Dante to enter Hell, different from hearing about its existence, different from believing in it. Vietnam War veterans want us to grasp that being there was different, that they experienced something the rest of us haven't. You are changed. And you don't want to give it up. You *can't* give it up. You are changed.

A recovering alcoholic is, A.A. teaches, always an alcoholic. You don't get over it. I'm confused about the semantic rules for cancer. When treatment has been effective—partially or "totally"—do you say "I had cancer"? or "I have cancer"? "Cancer survivor" conjures up war veterans whose primary identification is with survivors of other battles, other wars, the buddies they eat lunch with at the American Legion, whose obituary portraits, however long they live into old age, will show them in the snappy caps of their uniforms.

Once an alcoholic, always an alcoholic. Once a soldier, always a soldier. Once mortal, always mortal. Yes, of course, my friend would say. We all have cancer cells in us; we're all mortal.

In this time when everyone rejoices for me, there's something I have to keep to myself, a secret I can't explain. I was glad to share my cancer and my treatment with old friends and new, but now—why do I not express more "yippee," one supporter gently complains? There's something I don't want to lose, something about death I want to keep alive. Perhaps, as Keats wrote, I'm *half in love with easeful Death*. I would be ashamed to tell you. What I need to know for myself is: am I ashamed of the feeling, or is it a rare treasure I've found and must cherish in my heart?

What you give up in the cancer time is the haunting of the past and the future. Those tiresome memories, tinged always with regret; those tiresome worries. In their place, a series of present moments—one buffet after another to the body, in the mind; the active work of discerning your reactions, choosing actions; receiving the offerings of people. If this cancer experience was dying—and in retrospect it both was and wasn't—it was more than dying; it was living in the present. Each dying moment, each moment of awareness of death, was a moment in the present, a moment of life. The moment of death itself, I came to sense, would be the most present moment of my life. So, yes, I'm drawn to dying. Because I'm drawn to living.

Certain intense periods of your life count more: living for a while in a city, taking a trip. During the cancer treatment time, nothing much happens, unlike traveling. One day is like another except for shifts that aren't flashy—a little more, a little less fatigue; mind a little brighter, a little duller. Then there are the markers—the days of chemotherapy, the visits to the doctor. The markers are atonal, the days almost monotonous, the variations subtle. But you feel the presence of each moment more than usual. Each meal counts, as it does on a trip. Each strand of hair found on the pillow in the morning or still on the scalp, you count as a keepsake, you greet with whimsical friendliness, special but passing. A small house by the train track, laundry hung out, scrap of backyard evenly mowed, curtains closed over the glass doors of a shed. Who will step out the kitchen door to collect the laundry? This unknown person seems important, but the train is moving by and I'll never even see her, and already I've forgotten what town it was.

Certain years are like this, every moment important, even those I don't remember. The cancer year counted as much as sixty other years. But now I'm back to regular life. Days filled with this and that. None of it can be dispensed with, some of it is interesting, some of it is helpful to others. But these days can't compare with the simplicity, the intensity, the magnitude of days when I could hear each turning of the wheels over the track.

KEEPING DEATH ALIVE

. . . .

WHEN SOMEONE DIES, you want to keep him alive. It's not that you wish for a resurrection. Even the distraught young wife who walked New York from hospital to hospital trying to find her husband who was lost in the World Trade Center collapse said only, "I want to hold his hand." If he was alive somewhere and suffering, she wanted to be with him. She was not trying to wish him alive if he was dead. I once over-heard a sister say to her younger brother, "I don't wish for what I can't have." They were foster children who had been adopted; they could not have their original family back, and she knew that they never did have that family, the family they would have wished for. The people who were holding onto hope for survivors in the destroyed buildings were not wish-ing for what they couldn't have; they were wishing for what they could have—if they could have it.

The wives of the men who jumped the hijackers and crashed the plane in Pennsylvania knew their husbands were dead. They did not try to wish them alive again, but they wanted to keep their essence alive, their spirit. Their heroism, yes, but also something more delicate, more personal. The husband who had always said *Let's roll* whenever he needed to mobilize his two young sons who were dawdling. As his wife told this to the TV world, she smiled, and her husband was alive.

I was not really in love with death. Attracted, at times, the way you may flirt in passing with a stranger you have no ex-pectation of seeing again. Attracted the way a child is who says *You'll be sorry when I'm dead* and imagines gloating over everyone's sorrow. Or attracted because you've momentarily forgotten what makes life worth living and death seems eas-ier. But that's not being in love. You can't be in love with death, because death is not a thing or a person. It's not even a place, as in *I love New York*. It's not even a concept, as in *I love America*.

But death is a friend, and I don't want to lose my friend. Death is a benefactor, death is a teacher. Death made me more alive when I was deepest in the cancer time. Death made me able to give a little bit of life to people who visited me.

The danger is that now the shine will be gone and I'll be as dull as I ever was.

Where is there death in this moment? My Buddhist teacher gave me this question as a talisman. I rub it, I polish it, I ask it as often as I can remember to.

Though we walk in the valley of the shadow of death, we hardly notice. When we do notice, we have the habit of being afraid. Afraid of death? Or afraid of not being alive? I want to be alive now, and it is death—if I can just keep noticing, keep remembering—that makes me alive.

ANGER AND DEPRESSION

. . . .

"If you wish to move your reader,"
Chekhov wrote, "you must write more coldly."

—JANE HIRSHFIELD, "In Praise of Coldness"

I JOIN THE mayor and another townsperson after a meeting. In the middle of our conversation about town matters, the mayor suddenly asks me, "You never got depressed?"

"No, I really didn't," I say, almost apologetically.

"That's amazing."

We go on with our conversation about town matters.

I've noticed before that the mayor watches me, as you might watch a bright child you are fond of in a spelling bee. Will she suddenly miss? Will it be a word she should have known? Will it be a word no one has ever heard of? Why does a child want to do this anyway, instead of soccer?

People expect certain responses in a cancer patient. One is depression. Another is anger. A friend says, "I remember your anger when you were sorting your father's belongings." I am startled by the degree of my failure to communicate to her what I had really felt, what the point of my story was.

My father died two days after I got the news I was likely to have advanced cancer. When I was clearing out his apartment, sorting through his many files and piles of papers, I found it easy to discard large amounts of material I might have deliberated over in another year. The principle was: if the only person interested in this is me, then it can be tossed, because *I won't be here.* Every time I began to get tired of the process and lose my perspective, I would remind myself, *I won't be here,* and it would become easy again. I saved some papers related to my father's time working with F.D.R. because my son, not I, might be interested. I felt wonderfully free. When I had dismantled other parental homes—my father's at an earlier move, my parents'-in-law—the process had been a struggle: what to keep, for whom, how, why. This time it was simple. It seemed like a model for other aspects of life. Keeping things, attachment: none of that mattered, because *I won't be here.* I felt emancipated.

When my friend said, "I remember your anger," I made myself pause and consider. Could I have been fooling myself? Was she seeing anger I was unaware of? It's tiring to dismantle things. It's sad when your father dies. It's troubling to know that you are going to die. But no, it was not anger. It was almost gaiety. I had the rare feeling that I knew the exact value of things.

I can't expect other people to understand what I felt during the cancer time. What I felt was not what they think *they* would have felt. Their smile, their kind look when I tried to tell them what I was feeling—these came from their sympathy, their concern for me, not necessarily their understanding.

Even people who have or have had cancer do not necessarily feel what I felt. "He shouldn't have told you that," a cancer friend says to me about some stark information the doctor passed on to me. I don't agree at all. I would hate having information withheld from me. The wife of another cancer friend says, "I didn't ask how long my husband had to live. I didn't want to know." Some parents-to-be don't want to be told the sex of their baby. My feeling was: if someone else knows the sex of my baby, why shouldn't I know? I like secrets, but I don't like other people knowing my secret when I don't.

WHY DID I not feel anger or depression? I had felt those emotions before and I've felt them since. It was as if they slunk out to the shed the day cancer became my live-in partner.

Jane Hirshfield, exploring Chekhov's advice to "write more coldly," discovers a "preserving dispassion" in the work of Chekhov and others. This phrase casts light on why I had no time for anger or depression. I was busy preserving—not some specific past of my own or my father's, not some tomorrow I couldn't imagine. I wanted to preserve the moment I was in, and only for that moment—a delicate operation since each moment passes to the next. I didn't want to be diverted by the passions, such as anger, or by death-in-life, which is depression. Some atavistic instinct was aroused suddenly by the change in my situation, as my half-blind-and-deaf old cat's instinct of alertness is aroused by something she senses, a change in her environment, a flicker of shadow.

People look for anger and depression because those are feelings they know, feelings they can imagine. People in our government look for recognizable behavior among the Pashtuns of Afghanistan, not realizing that where the culture is different the responses will be unfamiliar. The starting point for Pashtun reactions, I heard on NPR, is "Pashtun honor": a tiny slight—someone looks at your daughter wrong—can lead to a grudge held for many generations. The starting point for people who don't have cancer is an assumption that they will live forever, or at least for an unforeseeably long time. Some people near death want to hold onto this earlier culture, the assumptions they used to live by. But sometimes you see an old person who seems calmer than he used to be. This may be someone who has recognized his own mortality, who doesn't have time for anger or depression because he's busy being alive for that moment.

BOTH ANGER AND depression have now slunk back into my house from the shed, since cancer has moved out. I'm disappointed. I learned what it was like to have no room for anger and depression, so why are they here again?

They're here again because there is room for them again. I've returned to the old hard work of trying to live right. Cancer's not here to help me anymore. The memory is still with me, though, and sometimes that helps but sometimes it makes things worse. We recently had repairs done on our house, which took more time than we wanted and kept us from concentrating on other things. When the contractor arrived one day and said, with urgency, that there was still more work to be done, anger filled me. *You have assaulted me, you have robbed me*, my anger said. *My money*—always a symbol, of course—*and my time, two months of my precious time: you have taken them, and now you insist on more.* And, pressing behind anger, depression said: *I'm not living the way I want, the way I promised myself to live, and I don't know how long I have.*

Life has returned to normal, you could say. The contractor was hard-sell, which has always tried my equanimity. Cancer took me out of the normal, lifted me above the mundane.

But it's more than that. Cancer set a high standard. Life was actually better then—more intense, more noble, more immediate. A performance was demanded of me and I did pretty well. People complimented me. I went to bed at night feeling satisfied with the work of the day. It was a kind of high, and now I'm rebounding. Well, there were drugs involved, in fact, and I'm off them now.

I can't keep it up, with cancer not here to help, but I remember what it was like. I know that the only one who can do the living is me, so when something from outside threatens what I know—the pushy contractor—I move against that outside threat with anger. And I move against my inside disappointment and shame with depression. Anger and depression have a strong life force of their own. They hide like microscopic cancer cells, biding their time. Like Edgar in *King Lear,* they *lurk, lurk.*

All this would be a bit much to explain to the mayor. I barely understand it myself.

LA DIRITTA VIA ERA SMARRITA

· ·

> The past is a foreign country: they do things differently there.
> —L.P. HARTLEY, *The Go-Between*

WHY DO WE feel off-balance when we project ourselves into a memory, even a memory of a year ago, a few months ago? We reread an old letter, we hear an evocative song, and we're back in an earlier time; but it's a foreign country, now no longer what it was then. We're in a different present now, and our symbolic interpretation has changed.

Five days before the World Trade Center disaster, I dreamed I was walking through a barren city scene, a hillside of streets, sidewalks, low buildings, no trees. It was early morning, but the sky was extremely dark in a beautifully dramatic way, a study in browns, lurid light, like certain Baroque Dutch landscapes. It was a dream version of Beacon Hill in Boston. I realized I was barefoot. Taking a shortcut across the hill, I passed children lying on the sidewalk in pairs, hugging each other for comfort or for warmth as they slept. I decided I would go to my friend Marilyn's and knock on the door, though I was unexpected, for breakfast.

Coming out of this dream, I felt uneasy, vulnerable. What awakened me was a strange unidentifiable sound boring into my subconscious. It might be an insect chorus rhythmically churning. Actually the outside walls of the school next door were being scoured by some huge cleaning device. The ambiguity of the sound enveloping me as I shifted from sleep to waking felt threatening. Was I surrounded by a wonderful rich sound of nature or by something mechanical, alien? In either case, there was no escaping it.

THAT DISTURBING SOUND and the dream seemed like the limbo time of cancer I was in. Nothing was wrong—I was walking freely, I could explore a city—but there were suggestions of danger: the sky though beautiful was dark, the sleeping children were actually homeless, my feet were unprotected as I walked. The sound I couldn't avoid hearing might be the caress of nature or the assault of a machine. As with cancer, as with life, solace was the possibility of knocking on a friend's door for breakfast.

After September 11, I learned that many had had premonitory dreams. Certainly mine could have been one—the bleak cityscape that looked war-torn, the lost children—but obviously I couldn't have understood it as a premonition before September 11. Seeing the dream from a new present gave it a new look.

A few days before that dream, I recorded another with familiar elements. I was in Parrish Hall (or a dream version of it), the huge all-purpose granite building I had lived in when a student at Swarthmore. Although my room had been on the fourth floor, now the staircase was blocked off because of disrepair above the second floor. When I left the building, late to meet someone, I had to make a wide circle around the campus because there was no direct way to where I was going. The first road I came to went up at a very steep angle—too steep, I thought—and I went on, looking for another way.

Nel mezzo del cammin di nostra vita
mi ritrovai per una selva oscura,
che la diritta via era smarrita.

(In the middle of our life's journey
I found myself in a dark wood,
where the straight way was covered over.)

—DANTE, *Inferno*

The complex old building. . . late. . . trying to find the way. I dream such images often. But because of my lung cancer, my thought was: "These ways that are steep—stairs, roads—that will require extra breath and strength in the lungs, are either blocked off or seem too challenging to me." Symbols become the body. The body becomes symbols.

I rarely have nightmares, but I forced myself awake from one soon after my two hospitalizations for pericarditis. My symptoms of chest pressure were not yet understood as lung cancer. The pulse in my head was pounding, which might be why I dreamed of a watch, I surmised at the time. I had dreamed of a watch before but never, to my memory, of money.

> *My watch is repaired, and the bill is over $8,000. The bill is just slipped into a paper bag, I find it almost accidentally. At first I don't see how big it is because I'm not expecting it. Slowly my mind develops its reactions. Shouldn't he have consulted me before doing it if it was going to cost that much? Shouldn't he have considered the original cost of the watch? What kind of obligation do I have to pay it? Can I just give him the watch and be done with it?*

I was facing large expenses because of my two hospitalizations as well as home care bills for my father (who died a week later). Even so, I didn't think the dream was about money. "It may have more to do with the old theme of loss of control, and also waste," I wrote at the time. Now I think my dreaming self knew more about loss of control and waste than my waking self knew. My pulsing body was trying to tell me something, and it was using all its resources, including dreams. I did have pericarditis; my father was dying; but there was more. It's cancer, don't you see? All through the part of your body you breathe with and the part of your body that holds you upright. Do you get it now? I wasn't yet seeing "how big it is because I'm not expecting it." The dream signaled that the message had to do with loss of control and waste, but I didn't yet know that there would be—there already were—huge issues of value, the value of life.

SOMETIMES NOT JUST dreams but everything around me seems to be a symbol. My symbol, my symbol for this moment. Your symbol wouldn't be the same, and mine won't be the same at another time.

There's one red-gold leaf on the maple tree among the green. It is beautiful. Last year I was that one red-gold leaf. This year I'm one of the green. I watered the tree tonight because there's a drought. What matters is whether the tree survives, not the one leaf. For the leaf it's already too late. And it is beautiful.

Your maple leaf might tell you something different from my maple leaf. Or it might even be "just" a maple leaf, though I doubt it.

It depends on your point of view. The orange marigold blossom is covered by the long legs of a bright green spider. As I look, a fly lands on the marigold and the spider catches it. Bad luck for the fly, good luck for the spider, neutral for the marigold, strange and fascinating for the onlookers. Life is random, beautiful, unpredictable, and strange. Luck depends on your point of view.

I'm becoming tired of cancer. I think that means I'm coming back to life. It's taken a year and a half. It takes some people a year to get over the effects of anesthesia. Chemobrain, a study recently reported, can last ten years. I'm thinking about a trip to southern Spain. Until recently, I wouldn't have bothered my mind with long-range travel plans. It's hard, it's unnatural, to remember I may—still—have only six months to live. I can say it, but I don't believe it. Like the child who says, "I'll say I'm sorry but I won't mean it."

Cancer's been a useful symbol, but I'm tired of it.

I am tired of cursing the Bishop,
(Said Crazy Jane)
Nine books or nine hats
Would not make him a man.
I have found something worse
To meditate on . . .
—YEATS

I need something new to meditate on.

TEARS

. . . .

It is the blight man was born for,
It is Margaret you mourn for.

—GERARD MANLEY HOPKINS, "Spring and Fall: to a young child"

I AM WALKING around close to tears all day today. Yesterday I felt as if something was weighing me down, like a heavy blanket. When a friend called with some good news for me, I couldn't receive it; I burst out in a wail the reason for my sadness: "My cat has died."

Having a mortal illness doesn't make me cry. I did cry once—after our first encounter with the oncologist who entered the consulting room without a greeting and declared, "I know all about you: I've looked at your films." In the car afterwards, my frustration at the impossibility of communication with such a man brought tears to my eyes. The other thing he said—"The average life span for someone with your condition is twenty-four weeks"—is not what made me cry.

Every month a questionnaire is administered to me as part of my clinical trial. On a scale of 1 to 5, I measure statements such as: *I feel short of breath. I feel close to my friends. I have trouble sleeping.* One of these statements is: *I feel sad.* Usually I give this a zero, sometimes (to keep them interested) a one. If it were today, I would give it a high score. I feel sad. I feel sad about the death of my cat.

It's a sunny winter day. I want to look out to the front porch and find her sitting on the top step, soaking the sun into her thick gray fur. She was better than a thermometer. If it was a warm day, she'd find the shade. If it was in between, she'd be in the striped shadows of the railing.

Why do I cry over the death of a cat and not over my own death? It's simple. *I won't be there.* But I'm here now, and my cat isn't.

WHEN WE WERE quite sure I was going to die, and soon, we took Gabriel out to a nice dinner and told him the stark prognosis. "But I'm not finished!" he moaned. I held his hand and the tears came to my eyes, tears for his tears.

Gabriel needed me for himself, that was what he felt. I tried to tell him that he had me fully already, that whatever I was for him was inside him and would always be. A few years earlier, when we discovered that our old woods, where we used to live, had been logged, Gabriel wept and I wept with him. It was Gabriel he mourned for.

He was surprised to observe my tears one night as he sat on the edge of my bed and talked about the girl he'd fallen in love with in another country, the girl he knew he shouldn't marry, for her sake and probably for his. "Why are you crying?" he asked. I could hardly tell him. With a little help from me, he was taking a necessary step into adulthood. But I was left behind. The image of the lovely girl I'd never met and never would was in my heart.

I cry for what can't be. The ending of the story of Tristan and Iseult, the lovers who can't be together and can't live apart. The ending of *La Bohème*, when Rodolfo begins to see what everyone else already knows, that Mimi is dying. "*Corraggio!*" shouts his friend as the music swells with inevitability. Dido's suicide aria in Purcell's *Dido and Aeneas*: "Remember me! But oh forget my fate."

I weep for my cat because she didn't die the way I wish she had. I'll weep for my son because he won't have his mother. But—so far—I don't weep for myself. I have something to do, to live the life that I have. I'm busy with my task.

SKULL AND BONES

. . . .

... You could tell it had been there
from the holes in the clay and the empty place in the air.

—ROBERT CUMMING, "Deer"

METASTASIS OF THE CUTICLE

. . . .

I DON'T KNOW if Susan made this term up, but it came quickly to her when I told her, early on, I was sensitive to every twitch in my body. Something was amiss with a cuticle at the time. "Oh, that's metastasis of the cuticle," she said gaily. Amused, I resolved to be more selective in telling people about my little aches and pains.

Later my cuticle became infected. The oncologist said it didn't have anything to do with the chemo, which surprised me. I'd never had anything wrong with my cuticle before. He sent me to a regular doctor; oncologists don't know ordinary medicine, it seems. The regular doctor I saw, someone new, with greased upstanding hair (a current style), didn't shake my hand either entering or departing and showed no interest in my cancer. I've become very sensitive to doctors, not just to cuticles. He prescribed an antibiotic. If it didn't get better after the ten-day course, that would mean it was fungal and he'd prescribe something different. What actually happened was that it got better but then recurred. Through a series of phone messages (no actual dialogue), he re-prescribed the antibiotic. I chose not to get it. I'm slow, but I'm learning that I sometimes do better following my own hunches than doctors'.

Susan said soaking my finger in vinegar was the thing to do. I did that and it stung, so something powerful had to be occurring. It continued to sting but it didn't get better.

It's better now, although the fingernail is rippled like sand when the tide withdraws. What did the trick was tea tree oil, which comes in a dainty bottle for about five dollars and is applied with a tiny brush like fingernail polish. I'd never heard of tea tree oil. Are there tea trees? But I've become a pusher. Tea tree oil is a cure-all, at least for anything having to do with fingernails or skin.

Tea trees, it turns out, are eucalyptus. I did know about eucalyptus oil. In 1959, I was about to take a two-day bus from Nice to Paris, overnight through the winter weather of central France, and I had caught a cold. I dreaded the journey. The French family I was living with poured a few drops of eucalyptus oil into hot tap water in the sink, draped a towel over my head, and told me to inhale the fumes. That cured me, and my trip through night and chill was fine. One of my most beloved memories is walking through Paris in falling snow.

Why don't doctors know something so simple and available?

What doctors know is limited, about cuticles, about cancer. Do I have cancer still? Where is it? What's it up to? The radiologists can't see it. They can see all sorts of stuff in there, but it doesn't look like cancer to them now. It looked like cancer to them before. They've declared a *complete radiographic response.* But they aren't looking everywhere, and their instruments aren't infallible, and, besides, cancer can be invisible.

At some point during the chemo sequence, I had a lower back pain. I've had lower back pains before, but because I have metastases—I really do—in the vertebrae, my oncologist sent me for an MRI of the spine. The only way to tell anything about my cancer, short of going inside surgically, is with pictures. The MRI suggested that my lower back pain was just a plain old lower back pain. My body confirms that conclusion: the lower back pain comes and goes, just the way it used to.

In the process of learning that I was O.K., I learned a little more about the limitations of this technology on which I am almost totally dependent for news. The radiology report, while concluding there was no significant change in my bony metastases, gave different names to the locations of the existing metastases—now on the left side as well as the right, up a notch, down a notch from where they were before. When I got another radiologist to view the films with me in his cave-like inner sanctum, we discovered that the locations had been dictated incorrectly—the spots were still on the same side as before—but I also learned that radiology is a very imprecise tool. What looked like L-1 on one film looked like L-2 on the other, but they were the same place on my skeleton. A Total Body Bone Scan, on which suspicious spots glow warningly, is a rather small, dim image of my skeleton not big enough for me to wear on Halloween. How had the doctor known where to insert the needle for the original bone biopsy? If he'd put it in the wrong place, we would never have known for sure that I had cancer.

When I was at a cancer retreat, I met someone with an unusual kind of cancer that can crop up unpredictably anywhere in the body. One day she had a stomach ache and immediately took to her bed. The next day she was better. She told me that any discomfort alarms her. I understand. Even for cancer patients with a more common form of the disease than hers, this is how it is.

One doesn't want to be a hypochondriac. But almost every cancer story you hear starts with a person brushing aside some signal his body was giving. Often the doctor brushes it aside too. Tolstoy got this right in *The Death of Ivan Ilych*. That minor but persistent ache in Ivan's side was what killed him.

Being more aware of your body is a lasting legacy of cancer, one of the most useful. It's also something that happens when you age. Older people are repeatedly reminded of their bodies, of their mortality. The only significant variation is whether they talk about it or not. But what do you do with this increased awareness? Sit in doctors' waiting rooms all the time? I think awareness is the point, not necessarily medicine.

So one of cancer's lessons—that it plays a game of hide-and-seek—is accompanied by another lesson about awareness of the body. I pay more attention to my cuticles now, and I'm learning to pay attention to everything about the body. In fact, I'm learning to pay more attention to everything.

HAIR

. . . .

THE LESS INTIMATELY someone knows me, the more important my hair is to her. Today the bank teller, the librarian, and a cousin by marriage I haven't seen for a year all commented on my hair. My "haircut," they say. It's growing at its own rate (slowly) and in its own directions, beginning to crinkle but basically a buzz, like a new recruit's. The librarian said how lucky it is that I have a well-shaped head. Someone who hugged me on the street the other day kept saying how wonderful it was that my hair was growing back. Somewhat meanly, I said to her, "That's the least of my concerns."

I can say that now, but I wasn't willing to show the world my bald or my peach-fuzz head. I wore bandanas. My head may be well shaped, but I was actually a bit shocked to see what my skull looked like and how it related to my neck. My ears aren't as flat as I had always thought.

I went public in a series of steps. I planned to defrock my head at a Buddhist meditation retreat I was going to. Nobody there knew what I had looked like before so they wouldn't make studied comparisons, and it amused me that I would look like a Buddhist nun. I stripped earlier, as it turned out, because I was tired of wearing a scarf in mid-summer heat. I no longer cared what I looked like. Now I understand women with wobbly legs who wear shorts anyway. I started by letting people who dropped by see me *au naturel*. My recorder group met at my house, and none of them said anything. I took walks at night and enjoyed the breeze on my head. Finally, the day before the retreat, I boldly went abroad in daylight, right into the bank and the post office. It was done.

When you first learn that you have cancer and you are told about treatment, all the side effects seem very important. My trial drug had caused dogs' eyelashes, though never people's, to curl inward. This would be very painful if it happened, so I proposed trimming my eyelashes before beginning the trial. My doctor's reaction was somewhere between surprise and alarm. "I wouldn't do that," he said. Now I find it hard to believe I was discussing such questions with him then.

My eyelashes never curled inward but they did thin out. A friend undergoing chemo had no lashes at all and her unfringed eyes looked strangely naked. I felt sorry for her, and the next week I looked almost the same. I never noticed my eyelashes decorating the bathroom sink; it seemed as if one day they were gone, or almost gone. When I noticed the loss of my lashes, it was already accomplished, it was a fact, something I had to live with. A little like the fact of cancer: I didn't know or notice I had cancer; then suddenly I did, and that was that. When I was a teenager, I was quite fond of my long eyelashes with their natural upward sweep, though I don't recall anyone else commenting on them. When they were fewer and farther between, I was sorry but not heartbroken. I hoped they would come back and I wasn't sure they would. This too is part of the cancer story: when something happens, you have no certainty that it will ever change for the better. When the lashes came back short and stubby, I was glad but not thrilled. Maybe they'll be long and elegant again some day, maybe they won't. In the meantime, as someone at the P.O. said today because the weather is so delightful, "It's a good day to be living."

When people—especially women—face chemo, they think about the loss of their hair. To get or not to get a wig. I was lucky that my hair came out slowly strand by strand so it seemed as if it wasn't coming out at all, until the day I had to comb it across a bald spot like men I've always been a little critical of, and then another day when I realized a scarf would be a good idea. So chemo for me was not about losing hair, it was about sitting strapped into an electric chair as the afternoon light waned and winter darkness set in. That's how it seems to me now, anyway. It was also about the possibility that I might live this life a little longer. The people who were closely in touch with me during that time said little about hair; I think they were glad to see me at all.

Hair is not really important. And yet I admit I too have been obsessed by it, after, however belatedly, I began to lose it. I never realized how many parts of me had hair and how much my self-image involved hair. When people talk about "hair," they mean the hair on the top of your head, but the hair experience is much more complex than that. One day I noticed that my legs were smooth. My bushy eyebrows became pencil-thin. My pubic hair was so reduced I could touch skin preserved silkily soft like a baby's.

Then one day I realized my body was hairy again. Hairs were protruding from my nostrils. Now that chemo is past and I'm feeling fine, the daily growth of my hair, both wanted and unwanted, fascinates me and worries me. At what point do I shave the back of my neck, as if I'd chosen to have this "haircut"? Do I consider using an eyebrow pencil to restore the patchy lichen of my eyebrows to the look of their former shape and fullness? I resist. I want to be open and simply attentive to this process, as I've tried to be all along. No wig. No eyebrow pencil. But now I'm a regular person and my vanity—never totally absent—asserts itself.

I don't like the way I look. When people say I look great, I think: they mean greater than they thought I would look, greater than I looked at the worst moment when they kept their observations to themselves, greater than I would look if I were dead. I study my face in the mirror to figure out why I looked better before, or if I did. I study photographs. I keep on the refrigerator happenchance snapshots of last fall—after the diagnosis, before the stripping. One shows me the day after the diagnosis, my braid falling over my shoulder. I don't look too bad. Another shows me after I had my first haircut in thirty years, in anticipation. Not bad at all. There's hope, I guess. But without my old eyebrows? They seem essential to my idea of myself.

A woman at the cancer retreat telling her life story said, "Growing up, I thought I was the ugliest person in the world. Well, not the ugliest—there was probably one person uglier than me." I may not be the ugliest person in the world just because my eyebrows have no character, my head isn't perfect, and—the hardest to say—my face is now slightly fuzzy. I'm sixty, and I wasn't destined to look like one of the older women I so admire, with fine white hair loosely pulled back into a French roll, strong jaws, beaming eyes, and rosy cheeks. Would I rather be homely or dead? *Consider the alternative,* as they say. One forgets so easily.

I'm ashamed of the extent to which I've evaluated people by their looks. Perhaps I should evaluate them by whether they're alive. Or not evaluate them at all? I'm fortunate to have a cancer where all that's visible is my imperfect eyebrows. My sense of my own mortality is slipping.

. . . .

"A bracelet of bright hair about the bone"
—DONNE, "The Relique"

YOU MIGHT THINK that the death sentence would send you
into a tizzy of frantic activity, like a fly thrashing to free itself
from a spider web. I've found that my urge is almost the opposite—to reduce to the bare bone. When I was pregnant—
full summer in an un-airconditioned house—I didn't become
a busy nest-maker; I wanted to lie through the hot afternoon
half-asleep, on the old sawdust pile in the woods, or on the
couch in the living room with the floor fan blowing on me. I
dreamed or half-dreamed that the lotus of the world rose up
from my navel.

After my cancer diagnosis, preparing for another kind of
life change, I again wanted stillness, physical and mental. I
found it mildly interesting to observe the scientific method
in a research article a friend sent; for Bob's sake I made myself read about the advantages of mushrooms and soy; but
the word I wrote in my journal was *harmony*. "I'm just trying
to be in harmony," I wrote between my second and third
chemo infusions.

I began to meditate on the corpse, as Buddhist monks do.
Chemo, unnatural as it is, helped. A Renaissance philosopher
kept a skull on his desk. I had my own skull to observe. Since
I didn't lose my hair all at once or in bunches, I had the notion
I was somehow "different," as my doctor occasionally said,
tickling a little private pride. Ah, I was given my own way of
learning that I'm no different, no better, than any mortal.

*The head has so many hairs that if they fall out one by one it
takes a long time to notice the effects. Likewise any action, chosen or unchosen, unnoticeably at first, then incrementally, is*

seen to make a difference. Any habit, chosen or unchosen. Aging, from birth onward. Practice of anything: an instrument, a behavior, an attitude.

The skull was teaching me about life at a pace suitable to me. Quicker studies might receive their teachings with the loss of handfuls of hair instead of thread by thread.

I begin to see the pale skin of the top of my head, never seen before. The skull will gradually emerge. I'm seeing my pubic area for the first time since the hair grew there. I'm easing back to earlier ages and to my fundamental lineation. Skin shrinks and pulls into lines. Skin pulls away from eyeballs so the eyes begin to look more like sockets of a skull.

Three months later, I wrote that "I have become friendly with my skull." I discovered that its shape, always before hidden by hair, is not a smooth curve but has plateaus.

A child playing near the shifting shore of South Carolina found a skull—perhaps an ancient Indian—and brought it to her mother. Her mother used it as an ashtray.

The Buddhist meditation in the charnel ground invites us to experience the ugliness of decay, repugnance of the flesh. This is a useful exercise, especially for the young and healthy. But there's another way to look at bones, Henry Moore's way. When I encountered his sculpture in London, 1961, it was a moment of recognition. I *saw* something about the elements of existence I had not seen before. At twenty, I thought that I was like Edna St. Vincent Millay's Euclid—that I was looking on Beauty bare. Now I think I was beamed, before I was old enough to understand, into knowledge of reality, not just of beauty. Forty years older and post-chemo, I sit in the Hirshhorn Sculpture Garden, stunned by Moore's "Working Model for 'Three-Way Piece No.3: Vertebrae,'" a golden bronze monument to bones.

You are only bones, and your bones are the same as everyone else's bones, and your bones may be damaged (like Rembrandt's subjects), but your bones, your rudiments, are thereby beautiful. It is enough. Your bones, all bones, are related too to the bones of animals and to rocks and shells and coral.

Even the mortality of the Rembrandt faces I was so moved by an hour earlier in the National Gallery is transmuted by these shining vertebrae.

The light is cast on the face of the unknown gentleman, whose eyes show that he has seen sadness and pain, but the light shows that he—everyone—is blessed.

The light on the golden vertebrae shifts.

Sand is innumerable fragments of exo-skeletons. The nodules in my lungs are innumerable, my vertebrae T-12, L-1, L-2, and one rib are damaged. I sit at the table in the sunny window of the living room. A line of smoke from the healing candle Carol gave me makes a line of shadow on the healing blue Buddha Nancy gave me. I write the sentence and look again: now the Buddha is completely shaded and the smoke shadow is no longer there. Out the window a jewel or a water drop gleams on a distant rhododendron leaf. I write the sentence and look again: it is already gone.

I dream about a dream within a frame, a dream within a dream. I am in danger from enemies who have guns and intend to shoot and kill me, although there has been no provocation that I know of. I manage to escape them and am in hiding, but it is inevitable that they will continue to seek me out, will find me, and will shoot and kill me. I am waiting for this to happen, for the conclusion of the dream within the frame, but I get tired of waiting, so I decide to haul myself up from a deep place to waking. I don't feel upset or frightened because there weren't any real choices: it was an existing dream already in its frame; it was just a matter of waiting. I didn't like it, but I didn't feel that I was supposed to solve a problem or that I could still rectify a mistake.

The dream reminds me that, although I have evaded the cancer, eventually it will kill me. But the dream is about more than cancer, I think; it is about life—a dream that exists on its own, framed within a larger dream, into which one wakes.

I understand impermanence by watching the clouds form and disappear over the valley at Black Mountain.

Bob says that he understands impermanence by watching dreams.

POSITIVE ATTITUDE JACKET

. . . .

Positive
Attitude
Linen Jacket
Dress
Sale 67.49
Reg. 89.99
With firework
embroidery.

—NEWSPAPER AD

. . . .

> He would go to his study, lie down, and again be alone
> with *It*: face to face with *It*. And nothing could be done
> with *It* except to look at it and shudder.

—TOLSTOY, *The Death of Ivan Ilych*

I HAVE BEEN complimented for my "attitude" many times. I
modestly demur: I've had so much support, luck, good medicine, etc. It seems that cancer calls forth the mystique of Attitude more than other major diseases.

There are both positive and negative cancer mystiques.
The negative mystique goes back to when people referred to
the *C word* — something that shouldn't be spoken. Even now,
cancer is an uncomfortable word, like words for sexual or-
gans, a word to be skirted. "R. e-mailed me on Tuesday the
bad news." "You have been in my thoughts so often since
learning of your *illness*." "How shocked and upset I was to
learn of your recent *troubles*." "That *this* could happen to you
makes absolutely no sense." These are the words you use
when you write to someone with cancer. One friend didn't
know the etiquette: "A. and I were shocked and distressed,
Deborah, to learn that you have *cancer*." Who told him that?
What made him bold enough to say it? I must have cancer; he
has named it. I can no longer think of it as bad news, illness,
troubles, or simply "this."

Even doctors participate in this mystique. To me, *malignancy* is a malign, an evil, word; but it is preferred over *cancer*.

Tumor has a vagueness about it; sometimes it seems to function as a plural. *Your tumor has shrunk*: but I had innumerable nodules, so what exactly is my *tumor*? I have an *oncologist*, not a cancer doctor. Cancer is something famous people in news articles die of. Cancer is the subject of research. Cancer is a metaphor I've used myself: *She felt it growing in her like a cancer.* It's not just a word for a disease.

The negative mystique is avoiding the subject. The positive mystique is talking about it in a cheerful, upbeat way. Both are rooted in the fact that cancer is still not well understood. It seems like a curse, not an illness. My doctor may not believe in evil magic, but, "It's more of an art than a science," I've been told more than once, when I ask a question he doesn't have an answer for. When you're doing well, you're ungrateful if you ask questions; just keep on doing what you're doing. When you're not doing so well, you also need to keep on doing what you're doing and hope for the best. Once when I asked for a little extra information about my treatment, I must have looked anxious, because my doctor answered, "Let's have a positive attitude."

There are a lot of things people think you can do about cancer besides submit to whatever treatment has been prescribed — surgery, radiation, chemotherapy, or a combination. Books on cancer have subtitles like "A Step-by-step Guide to Helping Yourself Fight Cancer," "Taking Control of Your Fight Against Cancer," "People Who Conquered Cancer and How They Did It," "A Practical Guide for Those Fighting TO WIN!" The language is military: *fight, conquer, win*. The goal is to *take control*. Some books have a more narrow agenda, but *you* are always in charge: "Lifesaving Self-Awareness Techniques," "Building a Team," "Preventing and Controlling Cancer with Diet and Lifestyle." These books, even when they are about diet or exercise, are the sacred texts of Attitude. Studies have shown that people who have a Good Attitude toward cancer do better.

FOR MY WHOLE life I have questioned systems that give prizes for merit. The prizes I hated most were given for personal qualities, like integrity or school spirit. In school, having a good attitude meant you were working for a prize. I wanted to be a real student, maybe even a scholar, so it worried me that I might be striving only for recognition, rewards, rather than the thing itself—true knowledge, wisdom, insight, whatever. I respected people who didn't play the prize game. I complicated my life by pretending I didn't play it. A classmate in college once told me admiringly, "You're so uncompetitive." I'd succeeded at that game—appearing uncompetitive—but I was ashamed because I didn't want to play any game.

Some people think they shouldn't talk about cancer with someone who has cancer because they see cancer as a kind of failure. If I'd eaten right, exercised right, drunk or not drunk wine/tea, prayed, been good to others, I wouldn't have cancer. I didn't get the prize. I didn't even pass. The look of sympathy is sometimes a look of pity, or embarrassment, for my failure.

But there's a way out. If I have the right attitude even now, I have another chance to win. And if I don't win, at least I get a prize for attitude. Miss Congeniality.

This question of attitude is hard to track. When I took my several vitamins this morning, I felt good about myself. I was doing something constructive for my health. You could say that I was taking vitamins because I had a good attitude, or you could say that I had a good attitude as a result of taking vitamins. You could even say that the vitamins are more likely to help me because I have a good attitude when I'm taking them.

Likewise, do I score because I choose to do yoga? Do I get a better score because of the attitude with which I do yoga? Or is it possible that the yoga, apart from any attitude attached to it, is itself therapeutic?

You can find evidence for anything. My oncology-chaplain

friend observed a patient get better who had a very bad prognosis *and* a very bad attitude. This patient was such a grouch that even this chaplain wanted to avoid him. It was a mystery.

Getting closer to mystery is the gift of cancer. An e-mail acquaintance, the wife of someone with cancer similar to mine, writes about attitude but also about mystery:

> *B. has such peace and confidence in the Lord. He has such a good attitude. We are so thankful for each day we have together.*

The good attitude here is not about fighting, conquering, winning. It's about the daily thankfulness. And about peace, not war. This man chose not to do another chemo sequence recommended by his doctor. The previous experience had given him numb feet and flu-like sensations; not only that but his cancer came back. All he could do was live through the treatment. Now, I imagine, he can be peaceful and thankful and enjoy what's important to him. He is living in the mystery.

BALANCE

AT YOGA CLASS yesterday we practiced breathing through one nostril at a time. The teacher asked each person whether it was easier to breathe through the right nostril or the left. I said I couldn't tell. "It was balanced?" she asked. I assented. The right nostril's breathing has to do with the body, the left nostril's with the mind; the goal, I found out after I gave my answer, is balance. My neighbor on the mat, who is also my neighbor on the street, whispered to me that she was not surprised that I was balanced. She told me later that she and the yoga instructor had agreed that they can feel my energy.

I denied nothing. It is nice to be told that you seem to be balanced or to have energy, especially in the context of healing. But I wasn't honest with my friend. I enjoyed the praise, but it made me uncomfortable. That particular day I was in a bad mood. I did not feel in tune with several things that were going on. The yoga instructor, I sensed, was not as cheerful as sometimes, and this affected me. My neighbor had talked before class about wanting to "do something" about the terrorist attacks—maybe organize a parade with fire engines, get the kids to sell lemonade to raise money. I had found it impossible to tell her that I felt ambivalent about patriotic demonstrations. I was not balanced at all! I was repressed and irritable.

I am quite persuaded that yoga is a good thing. I love the awareness it stimulates, the subtle enhancement of every part of the body, the meditative pace of it. I am also convinced that breathing is—well, obviously—the key to life. It goes on without us, it keeps us going in spite of us, it has its own calendar for our life. Being more and more awake to breath means being more and more awake to life. Any little maneuver that encourages breath awareness is good, so I was glad to do alternate nostril breathing. But I balked at the idea, expressed as a fact, that one nostril has to do with the body and the other with the mind. For one thing, my nostrils happen to be shaped differently from each other. One is a nice nostril-shaped cavity but the other has a bulge that intrudes into the cavity and reduces the amount of open space for the flow of air: they are not balanced. My body is not symmetrical. Each of my breasts has its own shape, size, and personality. My arms do not lie on the floor in the same way. When I stand, one hip is slightly higher than the other. I have more of a bunion on one big toe than the other. My eyebrows, my eyes, are not mirror images of each other. To the extent that I have studied other people's physiques, in less detail than my own, this seems true of everyone. Symmetry in nature is wonderful, but so is asymmetry.

Balance is good. I'm all for it, and, in fact, I strive to achieve it whenever I can remember to. But really, yesterday, I just couldn't figure out which nostril was breathing more easily. I may have been distracted during the exercise, too, contemplating whether we should eat lunch in the cafeteria, or picturing the rubble of the World Trade Center.

Am I balanced—leaving yesterday aside—or have I fooled my neighbor? She has serious health problems and has two small children. She is searching for answers and wants to believe they can be found somewhere other than in standard medicine. Yoga, nutrition, herbs, meditation . . . My miraculous improvement is a beacon to her. She wants to believe it is my balance, my healing energy, that has defeated the disease. She wants to learn to cook the way I do.

So much in cancer and in other diseases like my neighbor's is a quest, a construction of beliefs. When I was in the worst pit of the disease, when I *seemed* to be over it, my well-wishers constructed for me a legendary positive attitude. This construction was effective: I tried to meet other people with a positive attitude, and this promoted a positive attitude in me. It's behaviorism at its simplest: the more minutes spent smiling, the better I feel. I see now that they wanted to believe in something—they had to, in order to help me. The more they believed, the more they could help me; the more I behaved as they believed, the more I was able to receive their help. I'm speaking honestly now. But I wasn't always honest when I welcomed someone at the door. I wasn't honest yesterday with my neighbor.

I don't know what balance is, really. Balance between body and mind, between the breath of one nostril and the breath of the other? When I think of balance, I think of how you deal with extremes. On a teeter-totter, balance occurs when two children find their relationship to the fulcrum. Walking a log across a stream, you hold your arms out and move your feet slowly, deliberately, above the abyss you fear only a few feet below. Balance is awareness, confidence, and—yes—belief. Belief that balance matters and that it can be achieved.

To the extent that I have balance, it is my adherence to honesty. Or—to be more honest—my effort toward honesty, my preference for honesty. There are some who would like me to tip one way or another. Toward science ("cancer is a defective gene") or toward prayer ("God works wonders if we only believe"). Toward trust in the doctors or toward belief in radical alternatives. Toward joy ("it's a miraculous recovery"), toward skepticism ("we'll see it again"). My balance-seeking instinct has been to try for the middle path.

BUDDHISTS BOW TO the Buddha, the Dharma, and the Sangha. One way to translate these Three Gems is: Awakeness, the Truth, and the Community of Awakened Beings.

I bow to Awakeness. I do not want to miss any precious breath of life. My health, my reason for existence is here.

I bow to the Truth. I want to know it, I seek it, I am open to it, whatever it is.

I bow to the Community of Awakened Beings. I want to recognize awakeness wherever I find it in all other beings and to acknowledge that, in their awakeness, they are a community, my community.

. . . .

MAYBE IF I'D lived in a town before, I would already know what neighbors are. I've lived in big cities. I've lived in the country, where I took daily walks seeing only occasional wild turkeys, deer, and my accompanying dog. Now I live on a little street with neighbors I don't know well. I walk to get my mail at the post office, to get books from the library, to get money from the bank, to attend Friends Meeting on Sundays and the Christmas Eve service and funerals at the Presbyterian Church. Christmas and funerals have begun to awaken me to an understanding of what neighbors are. As has cancer.

I've always heard people joke about casseroles. My parents-in-law lived in this town where I now live, so I knew the town already, or thought I did. How quickly people get the news that someone is ill; how quickly they appear on your doorstep with a casserole. My mother-in-law moved here from the North (more unusual in 1931 than now) and was rapidly learning how to be a new bride instead of a college professor. Two dressed-up ladies rang her doorbell. One said, "I'm Mrs. Black and this is Mrs. Gray. I'm deaf and she's blind, and between us we're going to find out all about you." This story is still told in the town.

There's less of a system now than there was then. People don't leave calling cards on certain afternoons. Sometimes I feel I'm a person visiting a remote country who doesn't speak the language well. But it's not a simple matter of North and South. It's understanding the way of neighbors.

We moved to this street just before Christmas five years ago. Someone from the street brought Christmas cookies and told us—a word to the wise—*the neighbors exchange gifts at Christmas.* The information made me a little uneasy, especially since I hadn't met all the neighbors yet. Was I supposed to give them gifts anyway? Such a gift surely wouldn't seem sincere. The first year I didn't participate in the exchange. As a newcomer, I decided to interpret the gifts brought to us as welcome-to-the-neighborhood offerings.

The next year was more tricky. I knew the neighbors now, but not well, and not equally well. I couldn't figure out what the Christmas exchange rules were. Having this lesson only once a year was awkward. I was becoming a fixture in the neighborhood at a faster pace than I was learning the culture. Exactly where did the geographical boundary of gift exchanges lie? Were the gifts to be home-made or could they be store-bought? Wrapped or not? Did one always deliver the gift, or could it be offered when another neighbor brought her gift to your door? Did one go inside and visit, or just hand the gift over the threshold, wish Merry Christmas, and depart? Was it correct to bring the gift several days before Christmas, or was it done only on Christmas Eve day? Was it O.K. to carry the bag of gifts from door to door, or should one pretend that one was giving only this particular, very special, tailored-to-the-individual-neighbor gift?

This year, five years into the learning process, I was still uneasy. I had learned the boundaries (no geographer would understand why the family on one end of the street is included and the family on the other end is not), but I was still bothered by the artificiality of preparing, packaging, labeling, and delivering cookies or roasted pecans to neighbors I rarely saw except when we were mowing our lawns in the summer. They weren't my most intimate friends in town, and I wasn't taking pecans to my most intimate friends.

I can't explain it, but this year as I, my visiting sister, and my son went door to door on the morning of Christmas Eve—I was the first to break the spell and stop worrying about whether the custom had changed this year (*Why isn't anyone coming?*)—I suddenly understood why we were doing this. I suddenly lost my shyness, my rigid commitment to sincerity, and felt happy to see each neighbor in turn. We laughed when we passed each other in the street with our paper shopping bags of cookies and pecans. I must have figured out the time to do it, or else I started a trend.

What I suddenly understood is that we were engaging in an essential ritual of being *neighbors*. Neighbors are neighbors. That's not the same thing as friends. A neighbor can be a friend, a friend can be a neighbor, but a neighbor doesn't have to be a friend. You can differ with a neighbor over who you vote for, where you go to church or if you do, whether you drink or smoke, how you feel about the school question—all things that matter in friendship—but you need a relationship with your neighbors, and that relationship is built on cookies at Christmas. It's a beautiful relationship. When I had my first Emergency Room episode that summer night, when something seemed to be going wrong with my heart, and the ambulance lights were bright in the street, one of my neighbors actually walked into the house in her nightgown (she told me later) to see if we needed her. During the following year, this neighbor would stop by, irregularly but often, with something she'd been cooking for her family and had made extra. Nothing fancy but always nutritious or soothing. Seeing her trailing up the walk in her apron always lifted my heart.

A neighbor who has trouble sleeping told me she looks out her window to see if a light is on across the street. It comforts her to know that another neighbor is up reading in the middle of the night.

Only a neighbor can walk into your house in the middle of the night. Only a neighbor can bring something that isn't even a casserole, and bring it without combing her hair first. Only a neighbor can be encouraged by a light on across the street. I certainly don't care what kind of cookies my neighbor gives me at Christmas but I care that she knows me, knows my name, notices whether my light is on or not.

The ones with children come calling on Christmas Eve with the whole family! I know they have other things to do, but there they are at the door smiling, all of them. I hardly recognize the children from one year to the next: I never see them. They are playing soccer, doing homework, going off to camp. But on Christmas Eve they seem glad to exchange wishes for the season. And the children have participated in making what they bring: tree-shaped cookies with thick colored pastes of icing, hard silver balls embedded in the paste. How is this different from the villages that fascinate me in Africa or Scandinavia? In my later years I have stumbled into something basic about human community, if only once a year.

There is another form of neighborhood that I have slowly begun to understand, late in life. It's called *church*. I was on the wrong track before. I thought, again, that church and friends were supposed to be the same. Fine if they are, but it's not essential. My tiny church, the Friends Meeting I attend, led me to this understanding during the cancer time. Quietly and without formality, one by one they brought me casseroles. Each in his or her own way. Sometimes a whole meal. Sometimes a flower or a thoughtful reading. Sometimes a visit, sometimes something on the doorstep. I know you know all about this; I'm the one who's a laggard in learning.

Cancer has taught me lessons that don't always coincide perfectly. That's life. The lessons of life—the lessons of cancer—don't always coincide perfectly. One cancer lesson is something about neighbors. But cancer has also taught me that I should spend my time in the ways that seem right to me. Making Christmas cookies for the neighbors? Attending meetings of my book clubs? Sometimes I feel I should cut out the superficial social actions. But it meant so much to me when L., from my book club, brought a jar of nasturtiums and left it on my porch. I wouldn't have known L. if I hadn't been in her book club, and I can't say she's a friend, by my strict standards. But the nasturtiums!

Book clubs, churches. Funerals. A friend from where I used to live said, "I don't do funerals." I admired her for this. She knew where her priorities lay. But now that I live in a town, I do funerals. When Bruce died last week, I started to go through my usual questioning. I hardly knew him—knew him only over the phone—so should I go to his memorial service? Wouldn't it look a little silly? Was it a good use of my time? But I knew the answer. It was the answer of the Christmas cookies. I'm a slow learner, but I was clear, finally, that going to yoga class was not a better use of my time than going to Bruce's funeral. A funeral knits the larger neighborhood, the neighborhood of the town, together. Especially a good funeral, as this one was, which spoke to all the circles of his acquaintance—his family, his colleagues, his congregation members, the citizens of his town, others with cancer, the wider human community. Among those the minister prayed for were "researchers." The minister was looking even to the future, not just the past, to those who might have the opportunity not to die of cancer, like me. I felt included, even though I hardly knew the deceased and was not a member of his congregation. I talked afterwards with other friends who hardly knew Bruce. They too had felt moved by the service. We shared this experience, as neighbors.

OUT MY NOVEMBER sunny morning window, I see two beautiful creatures. I don't know which seems more beautiful to me. The yellow cat appears from the grasses, noses deliberately along the path, stops and surveys, moves on, full of hope that a delicious bird will come into his clutches. Far above his head, a young mourning dove twinkles onto a thin branch, fluffs her breast feathers to the sun, smooths them down again, and rests, full of hope of being warm, of flying, for another whole day.

Hope. An old friend asks if I'm surprised at his opinion that "we" are correct in bombing Afghanistan. I think about his hopeless view that there is no chance for democracy anywhere in the Muslim world, that the only way to eliminate terrorism is through military repression, that the basic problem is religious fanaticism about which nothing can be done. But his question was specifically about our war in Afghanistan. I answer, "I'm surprised that you have so much hope." Hope that we can succeed militarily in a land where no invader from Alexander to the Russians has succeeded, hope that we will be able to penetrate a society, a language (or languages), a complex of cultures so different from those of our soldiers, our spies, our government officials. I'm really amazed that he has this hope.

But of course I don't really mean that he has hope. When I told him, thinking it would interest him, about the Aga Khan's plan to establish a liberal arts college in Pakistan, he said sharply, "Why would anyone want to do that?" I was startled. There are many questions about the Aga Khan and his plans, but this question is not the one I expected: why would one *want* to do that? I answered feebly, "So people will be better educated?" This is hope. He—at least in this territory—does not have hope.

One of my cancer phone-friends, the wife of a man with metastasized, recurrent lung cancer, tells me their doctor has now uttered one of the two famous cancer sentences: "There's nothing more we can do." The other one is: "You have cancer." Every account of cancer begins with that one. Both sentences announce the withdrawal of hope. "You have cancer" should always be followed by *but*. "There's nothing more we can do" erases the *but*.

She goes on to describe their interaction with the doctor. "He was cold. He has never been cold before. I used to think of him as warm." I don't know this doctor, but he's well thought of. He has become cold, I think, because he cannot offer them any hope, because he no longer has hope himself.

My phone-friend, in her own despair, forced the doctor to use more exact language. "So he's going to die," she said. The answer was yes. She talked to the doctor about the possibility of going on Iressa, my trial drug, through "compassionate use." For reasons she didn't understand, he was discouraging. She wanted to know if I thought she should pursue this possibility in other ways. Before I gave her my advice, I probed to find out whether she and her husband were ready to work on acceptance of death. Clearly they were not; they were mad. They still wanted to fight. What had kept her husband going during the last treatment was his notion that the unpleasant side effects he was experiencing must mean the chemo was rooting out the cancer. His wife realized this might not be true but didn't tell him. "We don't have any children. My brother died of cancer three years ago. He's all I've got," she mourns over the phone. I urge her to pursue the possibility of Iressa. "There's no guarantee it will work. If it doesn't, then you'll need to focus on acceptance of dying. But you need to know for sure that there's no other possibility." No other hope.

Another friend-of-a-friend with metastatic, recurrent breast cancer has just been told she will die within a year. They've run out of treatments, none have worked, and she's seriously worse. My friend wants to know if my trial drug may be applicable. A straw. A hope.

I see now how unappreciative I was when I was first offered the chance of a trial drug. I was told that the average life span for someone with my extent of disease was twenty-four weeks. I was annoyed at the doctor for phrasing it in weeks instead of months. I understood instinctively then, and more clearly now, that he wanted me to feel how short a time that was. The offer of the trial drug was an oar extended from a raft to a drowning person. Ungratefully, I asked questions about the side effects, about how harmful the drug might be. I believe now that that drug has saved my life, at least for a while; I am bemused by the suspicion I felt at the time. When I mention the drug to someone now and hear the skeptical reaction, "Well, I trust my doctors . . . ," I have trouble remembering that I too was full of doubts.

The work I was doing a year ago was quite complex. What I thought I was doing, and what I remember most, was developing a relationship with death, with dying. I wanted to live with death, as with a lover, before marrying it. I felt I wanted to start dying right away, not to waste any time. It wasn't that I wanted to die as soon as possible; it was that I wanted to *be dying* in the fullest possible way, by which I understood to live every minute of my dying. I accepted the prospect of death immediately. At first, before I was told about the twenty-four weeks and the trial drug, the possibility of treatment didn't even occur to me. I thought only of how to do the dying well.

When I was told about the chemotherapy I could have—its low rate of response, those who do respond live only a few months longer—and the trial drug, I chose to accept these offers of hope. Hope for life. So, at the same time as I was learning to live with dying, I was learning to live with hope. I suppose that the friends who stopped by with a flower, a digestible meal, an inspirational book probably thought my "wonderful attitude" had to do with hope. People who don't have cancer—and many who do—seem to define the work of the cancer patient as the fight for survival, as—even more than hope—the practice of faith. But I felt my work was to accept no hope, no hope for a longer life. In truth, I was doing both: living with dying and living with hope.

Sara hugged me with tears in her eyes. "Just because I cry a lot," she apologized, "doesn't mean I don't have hope."

But isn't it strange? Her saying that made me realize how little hope she thought there was. *Hope* has a *maybe* in it. It's closer to *wish* than to confidence.

Bettie said, "I wish I'd known you sooner." I knew then that she expected me to die.

There's something melancholy about hope. Now I realize that my old friend doesn't really believe we can bomb terrorism out of the Middle East. He just wishes we could.

PRACTICING DYING

. . . .

THERE IS ONLY one way to be born, from the body of a woman. If dying has the simplicity of birth, perhaps I can practice it, take Lamaze classes in dying. I am pregnant with my own death, and I want to rehearse the event. But birthing classes are based on the experience of all the women who have told their experience as well as those who have witnessed it. With dying, there are only witnesses. Tolstoy seems to have known what Ivan Ilych experienced while dying, but Ivan himself couldn't come back and give a report. So what dying is like is guesswork. Some students of the dying process have developed ways to be helpful. I talked to one, a therapist who told me she could guide me through a dying practice. But I didn't want to! I was stubbornly intent on finding—inventing—my own way.

As I moved into the time of charting my own course, post-chemo, I thought more, not less, about what dying would be like. Going to sleep at night I began imagining that I was going into death instead of sleep. If I did that every night, my dying might be as peaceful as going to sleep. Although I can't know what the time before death will be like—how much, in what ways, I will suffer—it seems very likely I'll be lying in bed at the moment of my death. So it must be like going to sleep, mustn't it? I know dying isn't always peaceful, but maybe I can influence my habits by learning to merge sleeping and dying, practicing every single night as I nestle my head into my soft pillow. Every single night, no matter what I've done during the day.

From my pillow I look into the darkness of a woods. In winter, with the leaves off, I can see one light on the far side of the woods. It may be a street light, but I like to think it is the light from a house, and I like to look at that light as I go to sleep, feeling connected with someone I don't know. Maybe I do know that someone, but in daylight I never think about it, I never bother to draw a line between our two houses. Looking at that far, consistent, steady light, I think of dying as going toward that light. And so I go to sleep.

The moon is full or a little past and the air outside my window is filled with pale light. I am merging with that light. And so I go to sleep.

The rain steadily tapping on the deck umbrella, hissing against the leaves, blends everything into one, heaven and earth, sky and ground. My spirit moves out, away from my body, into this full but permeable space, filled already with drops of water, with drops of air, with the pulse of crickets, and, here and there, the barking of dogs, like anchors, like trees.

I can't see the light from my bedroom window any more. Have the people moved away and snuffed the light? No, the trees in the woods have begun to leaf out, coming between me and the light. The light, visible or not, is there.

I am lying in bed in the mountains, facing a window that overlooks a valley. I turn my attention to a period of my life I've never been happy with, that I want to learn to accept before I die, to forgive. It is a dark period, and I radiate it with light. I let the light carry me with it, away, out, beyond. I am particles of light as they spread out into space. And so I go to sleep.

In the mountains, I look out the window at the lights of the valley; then suddenly they are gone. All the lights are extinguished! Has there been a massive power failure? No, a dense cloud has covered the valley, coming between me and the lights. I go to sleep whether I can see the light or not.

I blend into a mass of color, a beautiful dark blue, midnight blue, blue-black. Then it is gold-orange, the color that comes sometimes behind your eyelids. And so I go to sleep.

I immerse myself in green, a more difficult color to call up but lovely to become one with as I go to sleep.

As I close my eyes I see little pricks of light: stars, sparks. I am joining these manifold lights.

I am walking on a path of plush green moss punctuated by white quartz. Looking down as I walk, I see myself flying over the earth. I am flying over my life, my life is a passing landscape below me, an earthscape I know and am leaving behind in a joyous soaring, swooping, sweeping, wide-winged movement. I am awake.

All metaphor, Malachi, stilts and all.

—YEATS, "High Talk"

ACCORDING TO THE obituaries the other day, two people died "after a brief/long battle with cancer." I told Bob I would like my obituary not to use military language. I don't see myself as a soldier, and anyway I'm too proud to accept the idea of a defeat. A cancer friend recently said in an e-mail: "I hope the Iressa gets rid of those last little cells that showed up in the PET scan. Remember to visualize each time you swallow your pill and aim it right at those little suckers!" I had never even thought of aiming my pill like a missile at my cancer.

Proponents of complementary or alternative treatment for cancer often encourage the use of visualization, especially the warlike kind my friend recommended. Because cancer is a mystery, it is natural to try to use magic against it. Magic, prayer—whatever works.

Health is whatever works
and for as long . . .

—JOHN STONE, "He Makes a House Call"

YES, HEALTH IS a mystery too. An older man whose wisdom comes from living in the same place all his life and doing the work that came to hand told me: "All that is necessary is that you believe. Only a little bit. No amount of belief is specified."

I don't admit to my friends who believe in magic, prayer or anything else that I am low in belief. If I told them, they wouldn't understand, and they would worry (unnecessarily, unhelpfully) about me. When a friend assured me once that she knew I was a "good Christian," I didn't debate it because I knew she meant "good person." To sort out these terms with her would be too complicated, and it wouldn't enhance our friendship, which I value.

I DON'T DO much magic or much prayer, but I'm truly glad if others want to. I'm sure it's good for them, and it may very well be good for me. I feel relieved to learn that the Wednesday prayer group still prays for me; I was afraid they had stopped when I got better. There's no stopping them, because they understand there's no stopping cancer. I'm deeply touched, and my sense of being cradled by them helps me. The prayers themselves may help me, too; I don't know.

Visualization is somewhat different, because it's the cancer patient herself who is supposed to do it. It's less a question of magic and more a question of influencing your own immune system. But the immune system itself seems to be a mystery. We're looking at one version of the Attitude question: you talk yourself into feeling a certain way, in this case by means of imagery.

I was told that the Simontons, who developed a cancer-healing therapy involving visualization, first screened therapy candidates for their desire to live. If I had to go through this screening, I'd be caught between trying to present myself the way they want—eager to live—and perversely refusing to present myself that way, insisting on an honest neutrality. There are children who deliberately give wrong answers on standardized tests because they feel insulted by the rigid simplicity of the format. As a result these exceptionally bright children are relegated to classes for dummies. There's a danger that my resistance to formulaic right answers on the Attitude or Visualization section of the Life test will cause me to flunk the whole test. People less adhered to skepticism than I am would take Pascal's wager.

> Let us weigh the gain and the loss in wagering that God is. Let us estimate these two chances. If you gain, you gain all; if you lose, you lose nothing. Wager, then, without hesitation that He is.

—from the *Pensées*, #233

Cancer therapy is not the same thing as belief in God, I realize. But it too involves matters of faith. Pascal approached the question of faith by means of reason or logic. Cancer patients choosing any kind of treatment—or no treatment—are also thrashing around in a swamp of the unknown, trying to use reason but really making a choice about faith. As Pascal said, " . . . you must wager. It is not optional. You are embarked."

So people "have faith in" their doctors. People "believe in" visualization or prayer or auto-urine therapy.

I'm no different. I believe in walking. I believe in the power of friendship. I believe in trying to look things in the eye. And whether or not I believe, I am affected, sometimes powerfully, by certain kinds of experiences. I'm affected by music. Our friend Spence, lying on our couch for months after suffering a near-fatal beating in a Miami park, was certain that he was healed by listening to Mozart.

At a concert, listening to the second movement of Bach's Double Violin Concerto, I thought: this music is healing me. In intermission, Theresa came over to tell me: "In the second movement of the Bach, I thought: 'This music is healing Deborah.'" And so, surely, it was.

Several months later, listening to a recording by Perlman and Stern of the same movement, I noted simply, "the sweetness." And I thought of other sweet things. I thought of Missy taking her husband's arm under the umbrella to go down our wet stairs the night before. I thought of me dying, reaching my arms up from our bed to Bob, weeping in response to his tears, thanking him for the good years of our lives.

Music is powerful. So don't give me music I don't choose. I would much rather have silence than someone else's therapeutic music. And, if there are to be images, I need to choose them, too. I was so happy in the Boston Museum of Fine Arts, standing before Rogier van der Weyden's *Saint Luke Painting the Virgin and Child.* I bought a postcard of it and I continue to gaze at it every day, never tiring of the rich blue and green robes of the Virgin, the studious concentration of Saint Luke, the couple with their backs to us on a bridge overlooking a river winding toward the horizon. But in another dimly lit room of the museum, just before closing time, I became almost unbearably depressed by two great paintings: Thomas Eakins' portrait of a university dean, *The Roll Call,* and John Singer Sargent's portrait, *The Daughters of Edward Darley Boit.* The Eakins portrait shows the dean standing in academic garb, reading off names at graduation. Someone I might know, he leans slightly to one side, reserved, dignified, human. Inexplicably, the university rejected this portrait they had commissioned. The Sargent portrait was described by a critic of the time as "four corners and a void." It is large: a dark room containing four sisters separate from each other and two huge Chinese vases. To me it is a portrait of the aloneness of the human condition. I was so weighed down by these two paintings I had to get out of the gallery, even though I was sure I would find that night had fallen and that it was raining cold rain. These paintings are magnificent, but for healing or for dying it's the Van der Weyden I need.

A friend told me she had learned, through visualization, to have an effect on the flow of her blood. I can't remember why she wanted to do this—maybe to make the blood arrive at the spot where the nurse was sticking her arm to draw it out. There have been times such a skill would have helped me. But this same friend later had a breast cancer recurrence. She couldn't keep that from happening.

Cancer can teach you to have more control over your blood, your body, your life. Contrariwise, it can teach you the limitations of control. I wrote in my journal:

> *Just when you thought you were in charge, that you had it mastered (whatever), that reason and the world of light prevailed, inside you, in dark recesses of your body, something out of your control, unknown to you, was quietly, secretly declaring itself.*

I walk on the surface of the earth, oblivious to its curve, even more oblivious to the earth's interior about which we know so little. Is it true it is burning?

If I'd been given a different kind of cancer—or a different disease than cancer—I would have been given different teachings. What I was given is an invisible cancer, a cancer I usually can't even feel. I focus on body, body, body, and yet it's only what I think is going on inside the body. What my doctors think is going on in my body. They base their interpretations on—at best—images from the interior, guesses made by radiologists. Sometimes I get tired of thinking about it and want to put aside me, me, me. For the first time I've understood something of the Buddhist idea of the impermanence of mental sensations, the instability of the notion of "me." The more I'm pulled to focus on Me, the less I know what Me is. A friend recently wrote, "How's your body?" That's good: not "How are *you*?" Better yet would be: "How's your notion of your body at this moment?"

Sometimes I think there are only images, or that all we

know are images. And I have some choice about which kind of images I gather in to myself. If I don't want to bombard my cancer with military images, are there other images I'm more at home with? They don't have to be images of power or images of the supernatural. The Rogier van der Weyden picture doesn't have a single angel in it and no haloes. It does have water, light, and sky. These are my choices. And it has the tenderness of the mother, and the direct gaze of St. Luke, who records what he sees.

ANNIVERSARIES

. . . .

Already then inevitable,
the full collision,
the life you will describe afterward always as "after."

—JANE HIRSHFIELD, "Balance"

PARTY

. . . .

ONE YEAR HAS passed since I had my first manifestation of symptoms. I thought then I was just out of shape. I needed more practice so I wouldn't lose my breath climbing Crowders Mountain. Or I needed to recognize that the steeper trail wasn't for me.

A year later, we take an anniversary hike. Cautious this time, we choose a trail that doesn't go straight up, though it is a high one—starting from Mt. Mitchell, the highest point east of the Mississippi. I pant a little on some parts of the trail, but not more than other people, not more than I would have, say, two years ago. I want more! More hikes!

There will be other anniversaries, one after the other. The anniversary of the day I got the chest x-ray results that showed something was not right. The anniversary of the day I got the CT scan results that showed I probably had a malignancy. The anniversary of the day I got the bone biopsy results that showed I definitely had metastasized cancer. The anniversary of the first chemo treatment. The anniversary of the first CT scan that showed improvement. The anniversary of the first CT scan that showed "no evidence for recurrent tumor in the chest." The anniversary of the next one that confirmed the previous one. The circle of the year keeps turning.

When I got married, on the first of the month, I thought we would celebrate on the first of every month for the rest of our lives. When I had a baby, we celebrated weekly birthdays, then monthly, then . . . just once a year. How long will I celebrate cancer anniversaries? I want to keep on marking them. For a while, at least, I'll have monthly blood draws so my rhythm will keep going, like menstruation, like the cycles of the moon.

Before the most recent CT scan, I began to get a little tense. I felt a touch of depression. I expect this will happen every eight weeks, a few days before the scan. And then there's the period of a few days after the scan when I don't yet know the results. People accustomed to praying (more than I) must be very familiar with this time, when something has already happened but you don't know what, so praying is futile. Even the day before a CT scan, what's going to be measured has already happened. Even before last year's breathless hike, before the chest x-ray, it had already happened. That's what cancer is: something that's already happened.

You could say everything about me has already happened. A friend of my father's wrote encouragingly, "I know you are a daughter of the pioneers." If I'm a daughter of the pioneers, I have something on my side, something that's already happened, that my ancestors did for me. On the other hand, it seems I have a genetic predisposition toward cancer, and that too has already happened. These traits I didn't choose have been—what?—in a fight with each other? Or are they in a dance with each other? I choose dance. They will be dancing with each other until the moment I die.

I want even more from the anniversary than the hike. I've decided to write everyone a letter. It's a big job, getting the words just right to tell them how I am now and to express my thanks for what they've done for me. There are more people to send it to than I realized. But all this is important to me, and worth it, like doing wedding invitations.

I truly want to have a chance to thank people, especially the ones who sent one e-mail or one card many months ago.

Every e-mail, every card, made a difference and I want them to know that. It was all of them together that enabled me to go to sleep—as I thought of it night after night—"bathed in love." During chemo infusions I wrote the names of people like a litany, like morning bird song. When the I.V. needle was in my right arm, my handwriting was clumsy. Naming these people, one after the other, carried me through the hours in the chair.

Chemo #2: Prayer circles. I'm being lifted up by people in Jean's church, Rose-Marie's church, Nancy's Tibetan monks, nuns Carol has written to, and the Wednesday noon prayer session at the Presbyterian Church. Also the Bhatnagars in India and the Hopi woman who made the dreamcatcher earrings Margo gave me. A candle is lit for me by Susie Lawson and by Sauni Wood. My name is on a prayer list of Bill & Ruby Walker. People in touch with me by e-mail: Karen, Hannah, Barbara, Bobbie, Jean, Rose-Marie, Harris & Sheryl, and others. Others thinking of or praying for me: Margo, Irene, BG, Carol, Missy, Will, Ingrid, Erwin & Judy.

Chemo #3: Marilyn Rieger, Bettie Horne, Rose-Marie, Marilyn, Bettie Casey, Ralph Quackenbush, Ralph & Wendell, Margo, Marcia, Missy, Ken & Sauni, Susie Lawson, Carol, BG, Buck, Sally & Craig, Ann & Jim Mead, Irene, Taylor, Tony, Susan, Sheryl, Harris, Jean, Alice, Polly, Gordon, Jill, Deb Gibson, Doris, Judy Rainbow, Bassett & Liz, Barbara Tinker, Bobbie, Tom, Sharon, Larry, Barbara, Job, Will, Masako, Raghuvir, Carol Wilson, Jane & Jerry, Ingrid, Karen, Aron, Joel & Abby, Hannah, Bob, Gill & Siri, Connie, Anne White, Jack & Betsy Perry, John & Rosmarie Monahan, Fred, Erwin & Judy, Mike Martin, Maggie, Marge, Don Carroll, Patty, Ralph L., Ralph Pillsbury, Jan, Ruby & Bill, Bernice, Maggie Smith, Barb & Bill.

*Chemo #5: People give gifts in their different ways. Bettie
Casey—a knitted cap in her bright colors. Barbara J—linen
hat bought in Chile, scarf, baseball hat, gingerbread. Ingrid—
little pictures of me as Chemo Babe (bald and brawny).
Fred—a phone call. Lu Pierotti—a card, a book she likes.
Ann Mead—pansies. Lydia Smith—multiple cards. Prayers.
Unknown people praying: a mission congregation in the
Philippines; churches of Jean, Rose-Marie, Marilyn Rieger.*

They don't know how much they helped. A former colleague
I'd never been friends with sent a reproduction of a beautiful
Rothko painting—*Green, Red, Blue*—and the words "You'll
be in my thoughts and prayers every single day without fail. I
promise." This card had power. I want to let him know. At
the time, I didn't answer cards like that. I was releasing myself from anything that felt like obligation; I was receiving; I
was focusing on myself. Now that the year has come full circle (the first curve of the spiral of anniversaries that is coming), I want to be in touch with everybody.

But I know there are other reasons I feel compelled to
write and send this letter to so many people. People mark the
anniversary of a death. Why do they do that? Maybe it's to
say: I haven't forgotten you, my loved one, and I haven't forgotten your death, your dying, and what that meant to me,
and this year without you has been different from the years
before. Likewise, I'm saying to myself: I haven't forgotten my
encounter with death, with dying, this year has been different
from any other, and I don't want to forget.

That's not all. There's something else I don't want to lose,
and I am in danger of losing it: all the attention I've been
given. So this letter, if I'm honest, is one more attempt to be
loved, to be bathed in love. Then I can shift from need to
wish, move back into the old position where I'm no longer
the center of attention and may sometimes give attention to

someone other than myself. Even when the CT scan was just beginning to show "moderate" improvement, I wrote:

> *Sometimes it's harder to be "better." You perversely, guiltily have an urge to explain* — but I'm not well, you know, I still have a mortal disease, this may be only temporary, there are a few ways in which I don't feel quite myself but they're a little too minor to mention . . . *You want to tell about the "metastasis of the cuticle" . . . And do they thoroughly realize that this disease isn't curable?*

And when the CT scan was showing "significant" improvement, I wrote on chemo day:

> *I want people to keep praying for me. I don't want them to stop just because I'm getting better. Bettie: "I'll take my hat back."*

So what do I do now, when I'm well? All I can do is write the letter.

SOME OF THE PEOPLE who gave so much to me are giving back once again, and I love it. The colleague who sent the Rothko card writes now again, on another gorgeous card (Gino Severini, *Sea=Dancer*): "I've not missed even one day thinking of you and—just in case you may still need it—I won't stop now." This is amazing to me. This man who was never my particular friend is thinking of me every single day, in the faraway town where I used to teach.

I send the love letter even to a few people who didn't really qualify by sending me a card or bringing me a casserole. It's working! More love is coming my way. "You're an inspiration to me—your strength, courage, beauty, and spirit remind me that the world is full of terrific women who are achieving great things." Who is giving to whom, here? By telling me I have strength, courage, beauty, and spirit, she gives me those very qualities. I am suddenly stronger, more courageous, perhaps a little bit beautiful, and full of spirit. She says I gave her something, but she's giving it to me.

I'm not the only one hungry for love, for appreciation. Some people's eye goes straight to the hand-written sentence at the bottom of the letter, the personal addendum, by-passing or skimming the carefully crafted body of the general letter. One tells me more about the candle she lit for me, since I had mentioned it; another says I made her happy by telling her she had "lifted my spirits." Thank you for thanking me. We all want to be thanked.

I've planned many parties in my life but given very few. I like lists, lists of people, lists of names. Walking alone through a city as a young woman, I would mentally peruse lists of names for boys, names for girls, babies I might have though I had no partner at the time. Lists of names for characters in novels I wasn't writing. Later, vacuuming the house, I would concoct lists of people to invite to some celebration I was too shy to actually organize. Besides, my house was too small. During this last year sometimes I would imagine my funeral. I imagined it in places it would never really happen. I would imagine my deathbed scene, surrounded by people I would list in my mind. Really I want only Bob and Gabriel there. And I certainly don't want so-and-so, so better not to have anyone. But sometimes it made me feel good to imagine M. and B. and maybe N., all gathered round. The best plan I made was to fund a memorial concert (in advance of my death—like a "pre-need" funeral arrangement). The concert could occur after my death, but it might be more satisfying— at least to me—before. I saw myself sitting bravely upright in the front of the small chapel with my back to the specially invited guests pretending not to watch me while they were moved by the sounds of the woodwind trio or string quartet performing music I'd selected.

The letter I sent out was for a big party. Someone hosts a party (even a dead person), everyone else appreciates it, and afterwards the host (if alive) feels tired but pleased. People gradually forget it, but it was nice at the time.

We used to give a Christmas party, to which the same people came every year. After we moved, someone else gave "our" Christmas party, and people began to forget the original, the true Christmas party. We wanted them to remember it always, to say, "Remember how anyone who had an instrument played and everyone else sang, from those old paperback carol books you had? And remember how the children would go outside and play Blindman's Bluff? And how the finger food that people brought was always just right? And how the grandparents sat on the couch and smiled?"

Sometimes I say to someone, "You met her at our wedding." The wedding was thirty years ago and people did have a lot of fun, but Bob and I are the only ones who remember everyone who was there. Or: "You met him at Bob's father's funeral." Marker events, anniversaries, they come and go and become part of the well-worn fabric of existence. Half the people at our wedding, happy in the sunshine of my parents' yard, are dead, divorced from each other, or estranged from us. But the occasion! Daffodils bloomed so early in April that year.

Some people skim my letter and slip it into the wastebasket along with most of the day's mail. And even those who study it carefully, who learn new details from it, who notice some particular wording—I've released these people now from asking me every time they see me at the post office how I am. I'm fine.

But I don't want to forget. It's too easy to revert, go back to start, as if this year were a dream, as it often seems to be. Every day is an anniversary. *Hello sunshine!* With every breath, I want to remember to ask, as my meditation teacher advised me to, *Where is there death in this moment?*

> As long as she lived that ecstasy was going to be hers. She
> would live for it, work for it, die for it; but she was going
> to have it . . . She would have it, have it—it!
> —WILLA CATHER, *Song of the Lark*

TIME IS NOT LINEAR. It is the ocean, rolling in and out and
over itself, covering the same sand again and again. A piece of
worn driftwood comes to the top and sinks again and comes
to the surface again somewhere else and sinks below again.

Today I have a new doctor because my previous one has
left. Suddenly the examining room is filled with two doctors—
my new one and one who originally diagnosed me a year ago—
each thrusting out a hand and saying "Way to go!" They have
just read the reports saying I've had a *complete radiographic re-*
sponse. When I ask the new doctor how uncommon this is,
whether I am off the charts, he says I am close to that edge.

My doctor for the last year, who was young and perhaps in-
secure in his first real job, apparently never shared my unusual progress with his colleagues. And he was cautious in
giving me his own reaction, though he did finally hold out his
hand to shake mine and say, "Congratulations." With him it
seemed inappropriate to feel good about my improvement.

When I felt jubilation after the best CT report so far, I saved
it for when I was striding along the circular path at Jetton Park,
almost flying as I repeated, "She would have it, have it—it!"

I wanted to feel my doctor and I were partners in every
phase of my experience, but the better I felt, the less there was
to share with him.

> *He isn't interested in anything other than obvious cancer pro-*
> *gression. Not interested in side effects or in other aspects of my*
> *health, or in considering which details may be cancer-related.*

Slowly I realize I am saddened by this—because he isn't inter-
ested in or doesn't believe in my continuing health—and feel a
little lonely. He was interested when something might affect the
treatment—the chemo—as when I had a sinus infection and he
prescribed for that. But now, I'm history. At least until the pro-
gression, which he considers inevitable, happens. Then there
will be new issues of treatment.

So it's strange that I am now celebrating, several months
after the good news ("the reports of my death are greatly ex-
aggerated"), with these two doctors. Bob and I have a festive
lunch afterwards, at the restaurant in the middle of a shopping center where you can sit by an artificial lake and watch
the ducks. I love this restaurant where we've had a series of
post-doctor's-appointment meals. Today there is no new
news at all, just a reverberation from an event—a CT scan—
last April, again in June, again in August: a recognition by
two doctors that something special has happened. The
rolling waves of the ocean have rolled once more.

There is never any news. When you learn something, it has
always already happened. You get information you didn't
have before and you react to it. I don't know how I am until I
happen to hear something about how someone else is or I
learn something about my lung cancer cohort. I read and
reread the statistics about the high rate of death in lung cancer patients, like sucking a lozenge to get all the sweetness
from it. Today I asked Yvonne, my drug-trial coordinator,
what happened to the other people on her part of my national clinical trial. "You're the only one," she said, as we
walked down the endless hall to her office. "The other two
died." I pictured the one I had met once when our chemo
days coincided. She was in a wheelchair, in distress from her
bony metastases. Later I heard she'd gone to the hospital.
Now, long after it happened, I found out she had died.

Yvonne spoke casually. I'm sure at the time it was personal and painful for her, but now it was a fact from her study. I could have been one of the ones who died.

SMALL

. . . .

SEPTEMBER 11: another anniversary, but this one, in the sea roll of time, becomes ground zero for anniversaries of the future. Other people's anniversaries, the world's.

On September 11, 2000, I was having my original CT scan. The technician came in, looking a little surprised, as I was lying on the gurney that wheeled me in and out of the circling machine and in and out again. "Have you ever had cancer?" she asked. I said no but I had had a breast biopsy once. "Oh, maybe that's what I'm seeing." Why did she ask? It was just something she had to ask, she said, for the radiologist. I suspected that she was seeing something quite abnormal, which of course she was. This CT scan was the basis of the diagnosis, eventually confirmed by a bone biopsy. This was the scan that made the cardiologist blush as he told me the results, that prompted my family doctor to call me on the phone. "Deborah, Deborah, Deborah . . . " he said, conveying more than other words would have.

A year later, on September 11, 2001, in perfect health, I am having a perfect day in a perfect place. Bob and I with our friends Rose-Marie and Bill are hiking up to Grayson's Highlands in southwest Virginia. It's what I call a Greek day— vibrantly blue sky, clear air, sunny and bright but not too hot. The slope up is just right—enough to work my lungs and leg muscles but not enough to feel out of breath or stressed. Cows graze the open pastures among clusters of jagged gray rocks. In a grove of small trees we glimpse a wild pony mother and child. When we want to, we stop to gather blueberries from shoulder-high bushes.

At the rocky top, eating our sandwiches, we can see in every direction. Lines of mountains behind other mountains. We debate which of the nearer peaks is Mt. Rogers, the highest mountain in Virginia. Smoke in one direction: a factory town? A butterfly. Two hawks. We're alone, as we have been all morning. I am completely happy.

A hiker appears over the rocky crest and we chat. "Have you been hiking since early this morning?" he asks.

"Not very early," I answer idly. "What about you?"

"I guess you don't know the news." He tells us a plane has crashed into the World Trade Center. And another plane into the other tower. And both towers have fallen down. And the Pentagon has been hit.

Rose-Marie thinks he may be a nut, making the story up. I notice he and his wife, who has now joined us, smell of marijuana. But I believe them. My eyes are out of focus with shock, and I feel a little sick. I continue to gaze out at the distant mountain ranges: I want to keep them in mind forever. The hiker points out that there are no plane trails in the sky. It is silent.

Reluctantly we descend, picking our way over the rocks, then past the cows, toward the car radio from which we will learn that the hiker's story is true. Not until the next day will we see the TV pictures, the flames, the smoke, the rubble, the weeping relatives.

Going down through the mountain meadow I think: *they can demolish the World Trade Center but this beauty is untouched and will always be. The world is huge and will not be destroyed.* When I say this to Gabriel later, he says: "Yes, it was not about beauty. It was about power."

No one was prepared. The reporters thought they would

be reporting other news that day. The firemen thought they would be putting out other fires, the police pursuing other crimes. It was said many times that no one could be prepared; it would not be possible to be prepared. Training for *disaster* did not encompass such disaster.

And so I contemplate my small story of cancer, a year later, an anniversary onward. This date will be remembered in history; it just happens to be one year after my little diagnosis. The slaughter of five thousand innocents occurred one year after my small death sentence. I feel how minor my story is. I imagine someone else being told today she has incurable, advanced cancer—being told this as patients, doctors, nurses watch buildings crumble and hear the shrieks of horror. When I was born in a Washington hospital in 1941, my mother felt she was not given much attention because the daughter of a general was also giving birth. What was it like for a mother giving birth a few months later, the day Pearl Harbor was struck?

There are events that are larger than an individual life. Five thousand lives are larger than one individual life. Death by terrorism is larger than death by cancer. A nation has been attacked. People are angry, people are afraid. I am alive a year after I got the news I would not be alive. It is a small thing, that I am alive. I took a breath just now! This is not news. I climbed a mountain. I ate a sandwich with friends. I saw a bird, a butterfly, a cloud. I drank some water. Even if today had been the day I died instead of the day I lived, it would not be news. This is the glory of it: that it is not news. That I have only a small story to tell, a small experience to analyze for you just in case you, with your small experience, may recognize something very small from it.

. . . .

There was a quiet, humble fluttering—small birds on
distant limbs. There was the pale hint of the sun against
his cheek, the smell of orchard grass. Ben became aware
of his breathing, and of the steady rhythm of his heart.
He became aware that he wanted to live, to have and
hold such things as a cherry orchard in midautumn in
river country. It was this world he wanted and no other.
There was no sweeter world he knew of.

—DAVID GUTERSON, *East of the Mountains*

I DREAM THAT the doctor I see to cure my cold is King Bhu-
mipol of Thailand.

No doctor can cure a cold, let alone advanced lung cancer,
but if he were a king? On the level of dreams, I must have a
strong desire to live, whatever efforts I may make to reconcile
with death.

After waking up from being cured by a king, I take a walk
with Bob and Gabriel to Sugarloaf, an immense sand dune
covered with trees where there is a bench looking out to the
distant Cape Fear River, blue and wide in the late afternoon
sunlight. To get there we take a long twisting path through
marsh, longleaf pine needles on white sand, black water pud-
dles we edge past, gripping branches. On the way back from
Sugarloaf it gets dark before we reach the lighted parking lot.
Between the pine boughs I glimpse the evening star. Happy
from the adventure of the walk, the special bench, I make a
quiet wish. I wish to live for a year.

One year later, in grateful ritual, we take the walk again.

What is this life force? It's just there, Rachel Naomi Remen
says; it's stronger than "you" are.

The Buddha said:

Being myself subject to birth, aging, ailment, death, sorrow, and defilement, seeing danger in what is subject to those things and seeking the unborn, unaging, unailing, deathless, sorrowless, undefiled supreme surcease of bondage, Nirvana, I attained it. The knowledge and vision was in me: my deliverance is unassailable; this is my last birth; there is now no renewal of being.

Reading this, I recoil. I think: This isn't what I want! I want mortality. I want life.

It seems I'm not ready to die. I'll practice dying, I'll try "lying corpse" as Patty holds my head in Reiki, but—honestly—I'm glad to be alive.

How strong the life force is. In *Schindler's List*—and this is just one of many examples from the literature of the Holocaust—a child jumps into the outhouse privy and finds other children already there, quietly standing in the stinking sludge. No one ever asks: *Why should I try to live?*

Perhaps the only person to ask such a question is the one who is ill and cannot recover. The further I've moved into recovery, the less I've asked the question. The life force reasserts itself.

I wake with the birds, happy I'm alive. When I don't sleep well or deeply, I still feel happy. Happy to be awake, happy to be asleep. My hair, growing slowly, black and white, feels silky as I smooth it in the directions it naturally goes. A few random strands of my old hair glint reddish brown from the before time. My doctors all have new babies, born since I've known them. Two ducks come near Bob and me while we eat lunch by the lake in the mall. There is a beautiful blue patch among their feathers. They settle down and take a rest next to each other. In our big house we too lie down next to each other for our rest.

I'm the way I was as a child. I want to be awake. Light comes, morning comes, and my desire is to get up and start experiencing the day. When I'm taken over by sleepiness, I gladly lie down and plunge into sleep. The adolescent wants to keep sleeping. The adult's mind says I need more sleep, go back to sleep. But the child sleeps and then wakes.

Thrush song coming through the window is as much a part of me as my thoughts. There's no difference between hearing bird song and hearing mental words. No boundaries. No self. The slow shock continues: I could be dead. The slow shock of awareness that I am alive.

PROGRESSION

. . . .

All that strange width of sea has now, oddly, changed in my mind. Uncrossed, it felt terrifying. Having crossed it, I feel as if I could cross it any number of times.

—ADAM NICOLSON, *Sea Room*

LULLS

· ·

Slowly we can tell each other some things about our lives:
runs, rests, brief resolutions; falls, and lulls;
hard, joyful runs, in certainty; dull, sweet
durances, human silences . . .
—JEAN VALENTINE, "Outside the Frame"

A SPECIAL DAY. An unknown radiologist with the ability to
interpret PET scans is figuring out whether the radioactive
glucose I was injected with is illuminating cancer in nooks
and crannies of my body or whether what it is illuminating is
something else. Or maybe it's not illuminating anything. The
reason it's a special day is that I don't know anything, can't
know anything, and can do nothing about it today. I have a
day off. No point in conjuring up scenarios because I'll know
soon enough. I can do other things. I can pay bills, just in
case I get bad or complicated news which will distract me
from paying bills.

Once I was a person who had a *partial radiographic response.*
A person who has received treatment, who has improved as a
result of the treatment, who is beginning to feel better because the treatment is over—but who is not cured. This person lives in twilight. Others are patting her on the back, looking for signs of joy in her, and beginning to act toward her as
toward a normal person. They believe that this is best for her
now, that this will bring her back to regular life. Cancer is no
longer discussed.

I have read that parents of a child who dies want people to continue to talk about their child, not to act as if the child hadn't existed. Therapists and advice columnists are clear that silence about the dead child is not therapeutic for the parents. I don't know if the same is true for a cancer patient or not: should people continue to mention cancer after the treatment? There is a danger she'll think people see her only as a cancer patient. When someone suggests that I am somehow vulnerable—might want to be careful about eating raw salad in a restaurant—I feel a little irritated. Then I wonder if that person sees something about me I don't see. I look in the mirror and notice the darkness under my eyes. I see a photograph and realize I'm not as stylish and healthy-looking with my short hair as I had thought.

A person with partial response doesn't introduce the subject of cancer anymore. She's alone with whatever she's feeling, whether it's hope, worry, or repression. It would be hypochondriacal to discuss cancer. It would be ungrateful. It would be morbid. But she lives with the awareness that she is not cured, that cancer doesn't go on fixing itself after treatment. Even someone whose cancer has been removed surgically must live with the possibility that at some unpredictable moment it will recur. Unpredictable moment, unpredictable location.

My luck got even better and I was handed a *complete radiographic response*. My cancer had gone on fixing itself after all, presumably because of my trial drug. I became a totally healthy person. I lost track of the idea—no fault of my doctor—that "we'll see it again." I believed we wouldn't see it again. I flipped from being a courageous victim to being a miracle girl.

Now I'm back in twilight. A subtle, intermittent pain in my lower rib is reflected as a *consolidation* in the lower right lobe of the lung on the most recent CT scan. Perusing the radiologist's report in the hospital parking lot, I know my reprieve is over. *Nearly stable,* it says. The several months of *stable* are finished. My doctor, too, behaves differently. In the past, I've had to insist that he look at the CT scans with me. This time, he plunges into the examining room with the words, "Where are the films?" It's only twilight, though. He isn't sure what the change means; the radiologist didn't characterize it definitely, just described it. We need this PET scan to produce an answer.

I have tried to stay in touch with my lower right rib since I made its acquaintance one day at the beach. My first note of it is tentative, reluctant:

> *I have some sense of strain in my right rib area. Metastasis of the cuticle? Stretched a little too much on beach or doing yoga? Always one can't help wondering: could this be the recurrence? I have so much hubris: why should I think this reprieve will last forever? We know so little about Iressa—maybe it can't sustain its power, its magic, beyond a certain point.*

I don't tell anyone about my rib until after the CT results. An hour after getting the disappointing results, I'm dressed up Renaissance-style playing my recorder at Christmas in Davidson. No one knows.

My journal becomes my confidant:

> *My "world" has shifted in the last week . . . I have reverted in my mind to being a person who is dying of cancer. It feels almost more oppressive—smothering—than before, because it seems more irrevocable: it's a recurrence, and the known treatments have already been tried . . . Also because I feel it. It's like the time when I had breathing difficulty: it seems real. Also because I feel somewhat alone with it so far. Am lying to others for the first time—"I'm fine" etc. when I really don't think so . . . Bob is reassuring people (the few who know anything)—why? To keep them from worrying? or to keep himself from worrying?*

I track the rib sensation. Later the same day, I write:

I don't feel the pain in my side. Maybe it's gone. Maybe the consolidation in the lung and the pain were something other than cancer. I feel like that other person again, the person I was last week, before the new little pain and the CT scan.

And later still the same day:

Well, it's not completely gone after all.

How I think about it is determined by whether I can feel it. When something is known only radiographically, it's abstract, intellectual. I think about "mortality," perhaps, or I make up alternative explanations. When I can feel that something, it's a very different experience. I'm slightly depressed; my mind, my whole being, feels clouded. I feel cut off from others by a constant physical awareness of something they don't know about.

By the next day, I've changed again.

No, it's not gone. But I feel better than I did. I've gotten used to it. Used to having a pain, used to being again on death row. It doesn't take long! So adaptable. Used to not knowing, to vacillation.

A reprise: an opportunity to review, to remind myself of what I learned the first time.

Even when there's physical pain, it's not the physical pain that causes suffering—it's the thought process associated with it. Buddhism talks about the two arrows: pain is an arrow shot into your body; suffering is a second arrow. You may not have any choice about the first arrow but you do about the second.

A new opportunity to learn. I've been chosen to participate in a trial, a learning trial. I am to receive carefully graduated doses of instruction. Mithridates, wary of assassination, immunized himself with gradually increasing doses of poison. In my case, I was given an opportunity to learn about death and life without, at first, having to suffer extremely. I learned a great deal, but I forgot some of it when I was no longer given the poison. Now I'm due for the next dose of poison—a little more potent this time, but still, perhaps, not deadly. Can I learn what I need to learn before being administered the final, death-dealing dose?

Two dreams of cancer. In the first, I visit a young girl I don't know who is lying on a cot, sick with cancer. We feel at home with each other, companionable. In the second, my family doctor, a very loving man whom I think of as a support although I haven't seen him for a year, is diagnosed with cancer, a fast-moving, deadly kind of cancer, and I understand that I will not see him again. I don't know what these dreams portend, but it's obvious that cancer is again on my mind. Perhaps my subconscious is accepting it. I am companion with other cancer patients, dying patients, and I will no longer have the support of a doctor.

I wake from these dreams into three beautiful moments. Gabriel on the phone tells of taking his morning run and crossing paths by chance with the Olympic torch runner: he was the only spectator, so he cheered the runner on. He is filled with delight. And there is an extraordinary insect on the screen door—a small translucent green-winged thing—looking in at me. And beyond the insect, on a tree in the back yard, a dewdrop gleams like a red jewel in the morning sun.

I am rediscovering the feeling I had often during the earlier cancer time, of acceptance of death and joy in life. The cycle is repeating itself. First the shock, then the acceptance.

I've gotten used to it. It was the shock of going back into Mortality that clouded me. Now I'm back in and capable of times of complete cheerfulness again—at the DHC board meeting, with

Margo at lunch, laughing at the thought of the New Yorker cover. Or are these times when I absolutely don't get it, am having spasms of the usual illusion of immortality that is the human norm?

There are two processes going on: my own internal process, of acceptance and resistance; the process of relating to other people and how I want them to relate to me. I've told almost no one yet—there's nothing to tell—but I begin to perceive myself in a new relation to others.

What one wants is either to be in real trouble or a miracle person free of trouble. In between—the maybe/maybe category—is the hard one.

I'm preparing for my next public presentation. I've been off-stage for a while. I note the egocentricity of disease, the permission disease gives to let one's basic egocentricity go center stage.

Come around me, bring me food and flowers, feel sorry for me, praise and admire me, show me that you think of me.

People who keep their aches and pains to themselves—certain old people, for instance—are true saints, or martyrs. I'm not like that. And yet—I don't want a replay of the attention I enjoyed before. This time I'll need more time to myself, more time to do some things I can only do alone. I'm preparing.

I don't want to waste time running after will-o'-the-wisp treatments, and I feel distaste at the idea of having chemo again. It just feels so wrong, to sit there and have this vile stuff, poison, drip into me . . . I don't want to lose what little time I have.

But today I'm not thinking about any of these questions. Today is a lull. Today I simply live my life. It's raining, after a long drought. It's cold, after unseasonably warm temperatures. The Taliban have been routed but Osama bin Laden is still fighting from his caves. The marigolds and chrysanthemums are still blooming. Even a black-eyed Susan has woken up under the grape arbor.

Thus shall ye think of all this passing world:
A star at dawn, a bubble in a stream;
A flash of lightning in a summer cloud,
A flickering lamp, a phantom, and a dream.

—THE DIAMOND SUTRA

CONTROL

. . . .

"Not to worry."
—TRAIN CONDUCTOR, London, 1961

IN THE SUMMER before my junior year in college, a teacher appeared when I needed one. As I handed my train ticket to the conductor at the entrance to the platform, he gave me the ticket to my life: "Not to worry," he said. I was amazed. He knew I was worrying. He knew I didn't need to. Although I continued to worry through the rest of my life, I have never forgotten what he gave me. My father, in the wisdom of his later years, said over and over again: "Don't worry, because you'll worry about the wrong thing." I worried about my heart, but it was cancer. I worried about the lower right side of my lung, but the place to worry about was in the upper left side of that lung. Cancer the teacher, once again. I can feel that place in the lower right, but the PET scan drew attention to another place, one I can't feel no matter how deeply I draw a breath.

The lull is over. I have the results, and they've been taken to the Tumor Board, the council of elders, and they have spoken. They have never seen anyone with my diagnosis do so well. Yes, there's cancer (probably), but they don't call it a progression. Again the images and the radiologist's interpretation of the images are what matters. The previous CT's couldn't discern that bit of remaining cancer; the PET can. It was there all along, when we were saying the picture was perfect. It's like something out of Mary Poppins: go behind the picture in the blue willow plate and other characters will appear, a more complex story will unfold.

The council of elders are "pleasantly astounded." My doctor says I've done better than "ninety-nine percent" of people who had chemo only, the only treatment there's been for patients like me until my trial drug emerged. This is wonderful news. But as I turn it around in my mind, I realize that there are different ways to read it. I have *only* a little bit of cancer; or: I *have* a little bit of cancer. The cancer is in *only one place* for sure; or: there are *two other places* that are less sure. Anyone I tell is very happy and dismisses the concern. I am very happy too, but I can't altogether dismiss the concern. I'm in a new round of the dance. The dance of death. The dance of life.

There isn't much I can do, except not to worry. When I got my original diagnosis, I told the news to a man I play recorders with. He said, "There isn't much we can do about it, is there?" Most people expressed sympathy or even outrage, but he couldn't help going to the heart of things. Of course, there are things you can do about cancer, up to a point— there are treatments, there are trials. But in a more profound way there isn't much you can do about it, and you really don't know what's going on. Even when you think you do, you don't.

The question of worry is the question of control. I like to be in control. I have considered myself a control freak, though not everyone knows this because I keep my behavior under—yes—control. Cancer the teacher: we are not in control. Much of my habitual worry (and it is habit) has to do with things I definitely can't control. I worry when Bob comes home late from an appointment in Charlotte. My meditation teacher pointed out that I was even trying to control the past, wishing certain scenes from my past had been otherwise. "I'm trashing your cosmology!" he hurled at me, trying to destroy the goddess idol of myself I had constructed. I want to learn not to worry, not to try for impossible control, because I don't want to waste the minutes of my life.

I can't control my cancer (that's my view, not everyone's). I can't control what's happening to my loved ones on the highway. But that doesn't mean I'm a victim, a person without choices. A dream offered me this understanding.

I am deciding whether to marry someone. Maybe I am choosing between two people. As I walk up an incline of muddy dirt, a path, I suddenly think: I could choose not to marry at all. It could be my choice not to marry. And I feel freed, happy.

This dream, I know, is not about my actual marriage to Bob. It's about the freedom to live my life the way I want. I couldn't control whether I got cancer, but I have choice in how I live with it, even in how I die with it. The arrow of pain is inevitable, but the second arrow of suffering is not.

It's not a question of appendix or kidney, but of life and . . .
death.

—TOLSTOY, *The Death of Ivan Ilych*

I SEE IN the paper that Bruce Jackson died on New Year's
Day. I've been looking in the obituaries for several weeks
now; one of his friends had told me it was "the countdown." I
worried about his wife, her long wait. I put on my list yesterday to write her a note. I'll write it, but now it's a condolence.

He has been a shadow, a twin, for me during this cancer
time, even though I never saw him. I got my diagnosis first, in
September; he got his in November. Like me, he had Stage IV
lung cancer, but his metastases were to the brain not, like
mine, to the bones. I called him when I heard of his diagnosis
and encouraged him to try to get on my trial, but he wasn't
eligible because of the brain involvement. Now he is dead and
I am alive. He took two trips to Europe during this year with
his wife and friends. Now he is dead.

On New Year's Day, before I knew he had died, I wrote about
him, my shadow, as a way of reminding myself of my reality.

*I know I may not have the whole year, and I may have only
this year, or part of it. It's hard to imagine that that residue of
cancer within my right lung could burst out, or that cancer
could appear elsewhere; that I could gradually lose—or even
suddenly lose—the capacities I feel now; that I could go into a
prolonged stupor or coma, as Bruce Jackson apparently has.*

As I wrote that, he was dead.

The reality of death, of life: so hard to keep in mind. Bruce
Jackson is dead. Does repeating statements help make them
real?

A friend who had not communicated since news of my "complete radiographic response" wrote recently:

> I read [your letter] from time to time and wonder: what am I to say to this? I just realized that all I had to say was: I am deeply happy that you are alive.

> I am deeply happy that you are alive.

And so he said it twice.
And I say twice, thrice: I am alive; Bruce is dead.

MY JOURNAL OVER and over again records the difficulty of keeping in mind the fundamental question of life and death. *The challenge has to do with keeping constantly in mind that this year may be my last.* How do I do that? Contemplating the ambiguity of my recent PET scan, I came up with a new gimmick: *Every day I will say to myself: I have six months to live. That will be a guide to staying on track. And one day—I won't know which—it will be true.*

My meditation teacher's mantra, *where is there death in this moment?* is a sort of anti-koan. If a koan is a riddle to which the answer is mysteriously hard to find, my mantra is the opposite: the answer is obvious. The answer is always the same, it is in the question itself: there is death in every moment. Of course. The action is in asking the question. But how to remember to ask the question? A slight pain in the lower right lung reminds me. But if there is no pain? I will waste the next minute, the whole day, just as I have always done.

Always. I have always made lists, always the same lists. New Year's resolutions, hopes, things I want to get done. The urgency of knowing I may die—I may really die—can help to get things on the list done. But then I realize that what matters is not what I accomplish but how I am. *What's most important, most urgent, is to maintain equilibrium, balance, presentmindedness, peace.* I wrote that this year, last year, the year before; I wrote it after the cancer and before the cancer. *We can only live in the moment. Sickness, old age, and death teach this.*

The difficulty is in remembering. I must remember to breathe. No, my body will breathe for me if I forget. I must remember to be alive. No, my body will stay alive for one minute longer if I forget. I don't control these things; I have nothing to do with them. I can yield to something bigger than myself. In fact, I might as well yield, because I'm not in charge. Cancer has taught me that I'm not in charge, if I can learn.

But that's not everything. Today, remembering about being alive and being dead, I tried saying to myself: *Bruce is alive; I'm dead.* Could this be true? Is that statement any less true than *Bruce is dead; I am alive?* Maybe I am dead, even though my body breathes, my heart beats. When I consider the question, I find I am not fully alive. Sometimes I think I might as well be dead. When I realize that, in a certain moment, I have made life worse for Bob instead of better, I lose my conviction that I should be alive. Why should I live if I'm not going to make his old age happy? When I realize that, during last week's snow, I didn't feel the ecstasy I've felt in other years, other snows, I wonder if I'm still really alive. What is it to be alive? My New Year's resolution should be: I will be alive as long as I am alive.

King Lear says, "I know when one is dead and when one lives." And so we all do. It is part of our human condition—our animal condition—to know the dead from the living, to recognize the moment "when we attend at the bedside of the dying and a 'person' vanishes from existence, leaving only a lifeless sack of flesh awaiting burial" (Jack Kornfield, *After the Ecstasy, the Laundry*). Sometimes that moment is obscured. The doctor summoned to certify my mother's death said he could still detect a pulse somewhere within her body and would have to come back later. Lear himself died thinking Cordelia was breathing. But death does become a fact. Bruce Jackson is dead.

The deadness of the dead, the incontrovertible fact, is a message available only to the living. But the living often give it the wrong interpretation. "The customary reflection at once occurred to him that this had happened to Ivan Ilych and not to him," and Ivan Ilych's colleague went on to his bridge game. We sweep the Christmas tree needles away, fret over tonight's meeting, put off reconciling the checkbook. Meanwhile the moon is going into total eclipse.

As the shadow of the earth—the earth we forget about even though we live on it—darkens the moon, the moon begins to glow. The solid earth's shadow, the solid moon's translucence, its roundness: we are aware of earth, of moon, fully, for a moment. And all of this light we are experiencing through the shadow comes, we suddenly realize, from the great sun, far away out of sight on the other side of the earth, the small earth, the even smaller moon.

The next morning when I wake up, I think: where is my eclipsed moon I had last night?

In the unmysterious sunlight birds flit about and the simple, rooted magnolia tree gleams wildly.

YOGA AND THE DEATH OF IVAN ILYCH

· ·

> "I have changed, eh?"
> "Yes, there is a change."
>
> —TOLSTOY, *The Death of Ivan Ilych*

I STAYED HOME from yoga because I had tripped over a board in the basement and smashed onto my knees. My knees needed a day of ice packs and gentle treatment, even gentler than Gentle Yoga. So Bob got to have a talk with the yoga teacher, Cathy, about me.

I had been rather proud of being (I sometimes thought) the most healthy, the most flexible member of the class. Why should this be something to be proud of? No reason, but one slips at times into the pointless old game of comparison.

It turns out that Cathy has observed a few things about me that aren't so stellar. My feet are crusty, a sign of poor health. My torso is rigid (although my nether regions are very mobile). And she's noticed that recently I don't seem to be as well as I did. Bob has noticed it too. He thought maybe it was because it was winter.

I had told Cathy that I had a little pain in the lower rib, that this corresponded to the discovery that there was still some cancer in one lung, and did she have any thoughts? What I meant was: was I right to protect the lower rib area when I did yoga stretches? But she rushed in with: yes, she definitely had some thoughts, I should go and see a holistic healer who is her mentor. When she told Bob I had changed, I remembered how I had felt awkward and tense when I asked her my question and how she had reacted. My manner must have communicated extreme anxiety and loss of equanimity.

It is hard to tell someone that you have a concern about your health, especially if you haven't been talking about it much. The pitch of your voice rises, your throat tightens, your eyes shift away from the listener's face in shyness, and sometimes you suddenly feel on the verge of tears. Sometimes you even cry.

How, then, should I respond to Cathy's (and Bob's—quite a different thing) observation that I've changed? For Ivan Ilych, seeing how his brother-in-law looked at him ("Yes, there is a change") affected the way he looked at himself. Studying himself in the mirror, he realized that "the change in him was immense." Then he overheard a conversation between his brother-in-law and his wife, who saw him daily. "Don't you see it? Why, he's a dead man! Look at his eyes—there's no light in them."

Some time after the chemo had stopped sapping my strength and my hair had begun looking like a living person's again, my neighbor, who had visited me regularly throughout, told me that the light had returned to my eyes. I had not known that the light was gone from my eyes.

An acquaintance told me my color had returned, that it had been awful a year earlier.

Have you ever seen someone and thought, "My god, he's aged overnight"? That person probably didn't look in the mirror and say, "My god, I've aged overnight." If I said to the person, "My god, you've aged overnight"—breaking a basic cultural rule—how would it affect him? I can tell you: he would age. He would begin to stoop, to shuffle, to leave his hair uncombed. Soon he would die.

There are countless stories (Rachel Naomi Remen tells some good ones in *Kitchen Table Wisdom*) of people who were holding their own but died the next week when they realized their doctor had given up. The meaning of this is not that doctors and others should fake their reactions and opinions when talking to a patient. That's certainly not what I want. But it is true that the perceptions of others are powerful. Literature can be powerful, too. It's easiest to see with movies. When I left the theatre after seeing *A Beautiful Mind,* I noticed that my gait was slightly off-kilter, like the gait of the schizophrenic mathematician in the film. I have almost nothing in common with him: I'm not schizophrenic and I'm not a mathematician. Yet I had absorbed his walk. I don't think I have much in common with Ivan Ilych either—I'm not a nineteenth century Russian judge—but, when Bob said Cathy had noticed a change in me, my mind echoed with *"Yes, there is a change . . . Don't you see it? Why, he's a dead man."*

I taught *The Death of Ivan Ilych* for too many years! Why did I feel it was so important for my students to read it? I used to give a class that may have swept over my students like a slight shift in the fog but to me was a powerful emotional experience, from which I always emerged dazed. All it consisted of was my reading to them every sentence of the last page of the story to demonstrate how Ivan went through eight major life changes—the numbers are pencilled in the margin of my text—in his very last instant, while the onlookers observed only his death throes. Why did I care so much? Because I thought my students, like Ivan, could lose their life over the placement of a curtain in a drawing room. Because I wanted them to see, sooner in their lives than he did, that it is never too late to make a radical change in your life, that seeing the truth is the only thing that matters, that how others see you is unimportant. And because I wanted them to have an experience of literature that would show them, even if only dimly, that literature can matter, that it can make your life more than what it was before, that it can help you see better.

Now, years after my students have sold their copies of *Ivan Ilych* second-hand, should I try to free myself of it (not possible) or should I try to understand it even more deeply in my bones? How others see you doesn't matter, and if you care too much (as Ivan did) it can lead to your death: "that drawing-room where he had fallen and for the sake of which (how bitterly ridiculous it seemed) he had sacrificed his life." And yet: how his brother-in-law saw him helped him see himself. "Why deceive myself? Isn't it obvious to everyone but me that I'm dying . . . " Ivan needed to understand that he was dying.

You can overreact to other people's comments. Bob is right: my feet are crusty because it's winter. You can overreact to what you see in the mirror, too. Thicker eyebrows are thicker eyebrows, nothing more—not a sign of health or inner well-being. Just because Ivan was near dying when his brother-in-law saw the change in him doesn't mean that I am near dying. But it is true that I am dying, you are dying, he/she/it is dying, we are all dying and there are messengers who pass by every now and then to remind us.

· ·

"Your beautiful pear tree."
—KATHERINE MANSFIELD, "Bliss"

LOOKING OUT FROM the deck over the apparently limitless woods behind my house, I listen—eavesdropping, it seems—to the dawn chorus, the first songs of birds that waken when it's barely light. Why have I missed so many dawns in my life?—I wonder, as I have wondered before. With this thought, I cease, momentarily, to hear the birds. But they are there, as they have been all my life and will continue to be.

The dogwood emerges from what I thought was darkness, presents its linear gesture before me, still, bright, modest.

And as the chorus fades with the brightening light, and I puzzle about the roar of heavy trucks in the outer world somewhere beyond my woods, a few birds still insist—a thrush, now—and Tiepelo pink clouds appear on blue sky between green leafy crowns of oak and poplar. I would never choose such colors! But they have been chosen.

I missed most of the sunrises of my life. Not all gifts given are received.

And some gifts received were never given. I was assigned to read Katherine Mansfield's "Bliss" when I was too young, too innocent a reader, to understand it. I sat in study hall one spring afternoon, with the heat rising outside the tall windows and girls around me scratching away at math problems or Latin translations. I alone was immersed in bliss, in the mood of that day and of my particular age, perfectly expressed in the phrase near the end of the story: *your beautiful pear tree.* That has felt more real to me all these years than what, quietly embarrassed, I learned in the next day's class—that the words were ironic, that the cool woman who breathed them was a false friend to the protagonist, she was her husband's lover. What my English teacher wanted us to understand—that the world can be treacherous—was one reality. But the words *your beautiful pear tree* stay with me still.

I have no idea why I've been chosen to have aberrant cells that are proliferating again with abandon. If I were living in another era, or even another place, I wouldn't know how near my body is to shutting down. With abandon I would be lighting the fire, stirring the pot, to feed my family for another day. Even now, I don't know.

EPILOGUE

. . . .

THOUGH SHE WAS known to deny it, Deborah Cumming was
a storyteller. I don't just mean that she could weave a good
yarn, but that she was adept at describing and reflecting on
lived experience—her own and others'. The essays found here
in *Recovering from Mortality* aren't conventional stories, after
all—they are careful meditations, observations of life and
death. So as well as a storyteller, Deborah was an observer—
and a listener. It was her acute observation and intent listening that enabled her to write these meditative explorations
with such convincing clarity.

As my mother, Deborah was a consummate observer and
listener. She paid close attention to the twenty-five years of
my life that we shared. If I had an experience on my own,
what legitimated it was coming home and recounting it to
Deborah: in our family, adventures or trips were expected to
be re-told sequentially and in full detail, a process that could
take as long as the original activity! Having listened, Deborah would offer astute feedback. I always thought most lu-
cidly when I was with her.

If I were to characterize Deborah's role in my own story, I
would describe her as the narrator. Beyond having a part in
the narrative, she was telling it. She made my life make sense.
It is hard for me, as protagonist in my own story, to carry on
without the narrator. It is a kind of loss that is hard to pin-
point, as no particular "piece" is missing—rather, the glue is
missing that holds all of the pieces together. I don't know
how I will overcome the loss of the storyteller in my life.

Deborah's presence—and now absence—as receiver and interpreter of experience has been particularly central to the lives of her immediate family—Bob and myself. Many other people valued this presence too, however. I was amazed and pleased to see all the people who came to the memorial Gathering in her honor, filling a large hall at Davidson College Presbyterian Church. Friends from all the times and places of Deborah's life: Princeton, Swarthmore, New York, Greenwood, Davidson, and beyond. In silence, those assembled listened to a Bach solo cello suite. Then, in the style of a Quaker meeting, individuals rose as they were moved to speak, each sharing something about Deborah as they had known her. Voice after voice, they continued for an hour and a half: remembering Deborah's service on the Davidson Housing Coalition, her recorder playing, her Indian cooking, her hosting of parties at the Greenwood house, her assistance of Laotian refugees . . . vivid stories that coalesced into a variegated but deeply felt portrait of a person.

Deborah liked to fantasize about her own funeral service, as she mentioned in these essays; having visualized a special event, however, she would wish that she herself could be there. For those of us at the Gathering, I think it was as though she was there. Never before had so many people who knew and loved Deborah been together in one place. The community of voices gathered on that day was the closest approximation of Deborah herself that there will ever be. I was deeply moved by the support of this community. Deborah too felt powerful support from many of these same people while undergoing cancer treatments. In the essay "Party" she describes how, to get through chemotherapy sessions, she made lists of their names.

Why was Deborah important to all of these people? I believe it was because, at some time, most of them had been listened to by her. Nothing connects you to a person like receiving their sincere attention. People did not quickly forget Deborah's interest in their lives. As a listener to and teller of stories, Deborah exhibited three qualities that continue to resonate for me: attentiveness, irreverence, and honesty.

Attentiveness. As has already been made evident, Deborah perceived and noted the meaning found even in small details: the tone of someone's voice or the peregrinations of a small bird in the yard. For the first eighteen years of my life, she, Bob, and I trained our attention on the rural South Carolina landscape where we lived. We observed the patterns of the place and its animal, plant, and human inhabitants. We tracked the changes that came in the course of an hour, a day, a year, or many years. When we left that home—the most wrenching separation of my life, prior to the loss of my mother—Deborah put together a series of albums about our time there, compiling photos, poems, journal entries, stories, and drawings. This document evokes our experience in Greenwood with such acuity that it transports me back there when I peruse it. For Deborah, everything that happened was worthy of attention.

Irreverence. Perceiving the genuine concern for others that Deborah evinced, people sometimes attributed to her a certain piety. Deborah was not reverential of any person, situation, or ideology, however—she could be critical in her frank appraisals of everyone, including herself. Some people may recognize themselves in some of these essays, and they may not always find themselves represented in a wholly flattering way. I can relate to this: I would sometimes come home from school bearing news of some prize or accolade I had received, only to have Deborah laughingly dismiss the whole premise for the award. This frankness did not stem from a lack of compassion, though—Deborah deeply cared about the people around her. Rather, she did not see compassion as being served by pretension. Her irreverence was tied, then, to her desire for honesty.

Honesty. Telling people exactly what she thought was not something Deborah always achieved—the truth sometimes seemed too damaging. She used honesty as her guide, however, and I always knew that her advice was sincere. Her cancer diagnosis enabled her to achieve new levels of honesty in her words and actions; if her life was soon to be curtailed, there was all the more reason to speak her mind now. I see these essays as the achievement of her most complete honesty: honesty about life and death.

The essays offer us a way of seeing and telling stories, characterized by attentiveness, irreverence, and honesty. This way of seeing has shaped who I am. It has been shared with the community of people who knew Deborah, and it infused the space of the Gathering. How many times can I say that I have spoken publicly in complete honesty? Only once, on that occasion. Now, through the publishing of this book, the offering is extended to you, the readers. The way of seeing represented here should be particularly helpful to those contemplating the prospect of their own death—but that can include everyone. Serious illness just heightens the sense of immediacy. Helping us all to quietly observe our own mortality is, I believe, what Deborah wanted to do through this writing, and in doing it we will continue her exploration.

—GABRIEL CUMMING

DEBORAH CUMMING wrote *Recovering from Mortality* during the twenty-nine months between the discovery that she had advanced lung cancer and her death. Born in 1941, she grew up in Princeton, New Jersey, and was educated at Swarthmore College and Columbia University. A lifelong concern for disadvantaged people led her to work in prison-bail, Upward-Bound, and community-action projects in New York City and Washington, and later in an affordable-housing group in North Carolina. A teacher of writing and literature, she worked with college and secondary students in New York, South Carolina, and India. While teaching in Thailand she translated and edited *A Premier Book of Contemporary Thai Verse* (with Montri Umavijani and Robert Cumming). She wrote short stories and poetry as well as essays; her stories are gathered in a critically acclaimed collection, *The Descent of Music*. She died in 2003 at her home in Davidson, North Carolina.

ROBERT CUMMING, Deborah's husband, writes poetry which has appeared in a number of magazines and anthologies, and has received awards including a writing fellowship from the South Carolina Arts Commission. He has taught at colleges in South Carolina, New York City, and Thailand. He grew up in Davidson, North Carolina, where he lives now.

GABRIEL CUMMING, Deborah's son, is a doctoral student in Ecology at the University of North Carolina at Chapel Hill. His research involves using ethnographic techniques—primarily interviewing and photography—to engage rural communities in conversations about land use and values. He has worked in North Carolina and Thailand.

NOVELLO FESTIVAL PRESS

Novello Festival Press, under the auspices of the Public Library of Charlotte and Mecklenburg County and through the publication of books of literary excellence, enhances the awareness of the literary arts, helps discover and nurture new literary talent, celebrates the rich diversity of the human experience, and expands the opportunities for writers and readers from within our community and its surrounding geographic region.

THE PUBLIC LIBRARY OF CHARLOTTE AND MECKLENBURG COUNTY

For more than a century, the Public Library of Charlotte and Mecklenburg County has provided essential community service and outreach to the citizens of the Charlotte area. Today, it is one of the premier libraries in the country—named "Library of the Year" and "Library of the Future" in the 1990s—with 23 branches, 1.6 million volumes, 20,000 videos and DVDs, 9,000 maps and 8,000 compact discs. The Library also sponsors a number of community-based programs, from the award-winning Novello Festival of Reading, a celebration that accentuates the fun of reading and learning, to branch programs for young people and adults.